I0123413

# AROUND

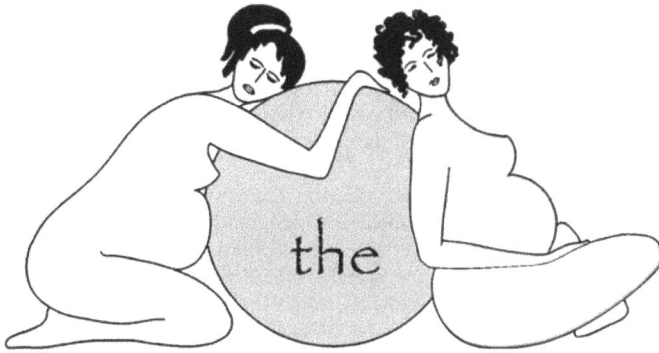

the

# BIRTHING

# BALL

by

Olga Breydo and Valerie Shor Perrier

To our contributors, our families, and our friends.

Copyright © 2011 by Olga Breydo and Valerie Shor Perrier

All Rights Reserved

Except as permitted under the United States Copyright Act of 1976, no part of this publication may be reproduced or distributed in any form or by any means, or stored in a database or retrieval system, without the prior written permission of the publisher.

This book is not intended as a medical advice, but as a resource of anecdotal experiences for expecting couples. Because the birth stories in this book have been shared from memory, the actual medical treatment received by each woman may have been more or less involved than what she chose to remember or share with us during her interview. While we have made every effort to ensure that the information in the stories, interviews, and glossary is accurate and reliable, we disclaim all liability for any unintended, unforeseen, or improper application of the recommendations and suggestions featured. We urge you to consult your medical professional when making decisions for your care before, during, and after pregnancy.

Please note that the names of all participants (except for medical practitioners) have been changed for privacy purposes.

ISBN: 978-0-615-38117-6

Design by Olga Breydo

Printed in the United States of America

# Contents

# Introduction

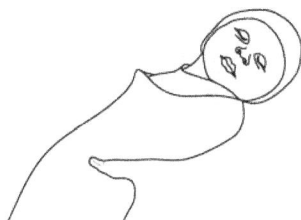

Congratulations! You are pregnant. We are glad that you chose this book, and we are certain it will be useful to you in preparation for your labor. So we urge you to read on.

We decided to write this book when we were both first-time mothers, amazed at the experience of bringing our children into this world. We have been close friends since our early teens and know each other extremely well. One of the things we are both good at is being prepared. Usually our organizational skills help us stay on top of things and ahead of the game. Interestingly, we both found ourselves rather unprepared for the birthing experiences of our children, even though we both felt we spent a good amount of time preparing for them.

We both successfully birthed our children, but the experience of labor and what comes immediately after took us by surprise. We felt that our expectations of what would happen were very different from what actually took place. On one hand we were stunned at the difference between what we expected and what actually happened, and on the other hand we were elated to realize that no matter how our labors went, our success at being mothers was definitive, because we brought to life our beautiful children.

Our goal is to share with you our stories, to provide interviews with medical professionals, and also to bring you the experiences of other women during and after their labors. Our hope is that as a result of reading our book, it will become clear to you that you should not be preparing for a *specific type* of labor.

What we mean is that labor is a dynamic process and can happen in many different ways, as you will see in this book. The best way to prepare for this event is to know as much as possible about the different ways a woman may end up giving birth and to be mentally prepared for any of these different scenarios. We feel that it is important for a woman to spend her time during pregnancy speaking to other women and learning about how they brought their children into the world, what kind of obstacles they faced, what they found most rewarding, and what they found most difficult. By exposing yourself to as many labor stories as possible and keeping an open-minded approach to how your own labor may happen, we feel you will be able to ground yourself in the ultimate goal—to have the baby!

As a result of our own experiences and our research, we learned that many women concentrate on preparing for a certain type of labor. Some mothers enjoy exactly what they had prepared for, while others are left feeling regret because they were not able to achieve the type of labor they had set their minds on. And certainly both types still face the challenge of handling a newborn—learning to juggle diaper changes, breast compresses, pumps, and sleep deprivation. Thus, we bring you our motherly advice:

1.      Keep an open mind.

2.      Learn as much as you can about as many types of birthing experiences as possible.

3.      Identify the practices of the hospital in which you plan to give birth. (Be mindful that different hospitals have different procedures for admitting and treating a woman in labor.)

4.      Educate yourself about what will be required of you once your baby is born.

5.      Identify your ultimate goal and always keep it in the back of your mind when making decisions before, during and after labor.

We encourage you to read through these stories with a pen and paper in hand. We urge you to write down problems that these women faced and spend time researching how you might tackle these types of issues should they happen to you. Once you are finished, you will have a list of questions that will guide you in your own research and preparation. You will be able to share this list with your doctor, midwife, or doula, and you will also be able to share it with your support team—family or friends who may be with you during or after your labor. If you come upon any unfamiliar terms while reading this book, please refer to the glossary at the end.

And once you are done, it will be your turn to tell other women how it is done. That is one of the benefits of becoming a mother. You will have created life, and will forever have the legitimate right to give "motherly" advice to others.

# Interview with an ob-gyn resident

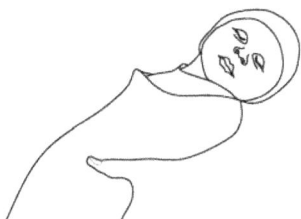

*Dr. Tunitsky-Bitton, is an ob-gyn resident, and has attended about nine-hundred births during her residency at a large tertiary hospital in Massachusetts. In this interview you will find her answers to questions about preparation for labor, pain management, a laboring woman's support team, progression of labor, and common misconceptions.*

*This interview is important because as you read the rest of this book, you will be able to flip back to it and draw a parallel between a situation during labor and how this situation might be approached from a medical perspective. Oftentimes, we meet women who are discouraged after their delivery because it did not proceed in a way they expected. This interview supports our theory that although there are many possible ways to deliver a baby, too many variables are in place to expect a specific result.*

*What types of hospitals did you study and work in? Please describe the patient demographic that you generally worked with.*

I studied and worked in community hospitals and tertiary care hospitals in Canada and the U.S. As far as demographics, I have taken care of people from different socio-economic classes, cultures, and races.

*Please talk about the importance of the birthing woman's support team.*

Labor is one of the most emotional, vulnerable, and challenging moments in a woman's life. The support group should know her well, meaning that she doesn't have to apologize for being moody. They should also be encouraging, and she should want them to share this important moment with her. This team doesn't have to have any special education or knowledge about the birthing process; that's what the medical team is for.

*Please describe which responsibilities you identify for yourself during delivery, and which responsibilities can, in your opinion, be attended by the birthing woman's support team?*

My main responsibilities include following the labor progress, taking care of maternal and fetal well-being, and deciding when to intervene. Once the labor progresses to the pushing stage, my other responsibilities are to coach the woman through the final stage, deliver the baby, and do any necessary repairs of the perineal tears. My responsibility further extends to taking care of the woman's postpartum to ensure there is no excessive bleeding and pain. All the while, I am also there to provide guidance, reassurance, and emotional support.

If my patient is someone with a high level of anxiety and low level of preparation, such as poor prenatal care, I will spend more time explaining, answering questions, and reassuring her. If she is someone who is alone, or whose support team is not helpful, then the nurse and I will play a greater role in coaching and taking charge of the situation. On the other hand, if the laboring woman is able to stay in control, her partner (or whoever is there for her) is encouraging and helpful, she seems to know the process, or she is simply a personality type that will ask questions when needed, then the nurse and I will be more hands-off and allow her to proceed and guide herself.

*Please describe why, in your opinion, a doctor may choose to schedule an induction. What are the right circumstances under which a woman should consider being induced?*

There are several reasons for a woman to get an induction of labor. Likewise, there are elective reasons for inductions, which I will discuss later. The most common reason for an induction is a post-term pregnancy. While the due date is based on the forty weeks of gestation, many first-time pregnancies go beyond forty weeks, often up to forty-one and forty-two weeks, which is normal. After forty-two weeks, it is considered post-term, and it becomes dangerous for the baby to stay in the womb, almost as dangerous as being born pre-term. As the placenta ages, less and less blood supply and nutrients go to the baby. This aging of the placenta starts taking place at forty-one weeks, and because the induction may take several days, it is reasonable to start inducing at forty-one weeks.

Other situations that require induction are indications that it is not healthy for the baby or the mother to continue pregnancy. These indications include inadequate growth of the baby, diminished fluid, hypertension, uncontrolled diabetes, and many other conditions.

As far as the elective inductions are concerned, many women actually request them when they are close to their due date because they are tired, have severe back pain, or waiting just doesn't fit into their schedule. Each provider has a different perspective on elective inductions. Some never do them because of the risk of failure and a subsequent C-section, while others gladly offer them.

In my opinion, it is very much case-dependent, but my decision to induce is typically based on the condition of the cervix. There is a score used by obstetricians that helps us assess if the cervix is favorable for induction. Based on a cervical exam, we can determine the likelihood for a successful induction. If a patient is about to have her third baby, the cervix is soft and has been two-to-three centimeters open for several weeks, and she also has back pain and other frequent irregular contractions, then she is likely to go into labor and successfully deliver with very little effort and minimal intervention. A first-time mom, with a long, thick, closed cervix, and no contractions in sight, has a high risk of induction failure.

*Please describe why a doctor may choose to start the patient on Pitocin. What are the factors that influence this decision?*

The main agent used for induction is Pitocin. This is the same thing as Oxytocin, which is a hormone that is released by the pituitary gland of a laboring woman to induce contractions and stimulate milk let-down. When the labor needs a jump-start, we start with cervical medications. Pitocin does little for cervical ripening, which is when the cervix becomes softer and opens. When Pitocin is given with an unfavorable cervix, the effect is contractions against a closed valve, which is painful for the mom and may be distressing for the baby. This is why most inductions begin with cervical ripening and take at least two days.

To ripen the cervix, medications such as Misoprostol or Cervidil are placed at the cervix to release prostaglandins, which make the cervix ready. Oftentimes this can induce contractions, and in some cases, even start labor without Pitocin. Misoprostol or Cervidil is usually given overnight in the hospital, and if the cervix is ripe by morning, then Pitocin is used. The Pitocin dosage is gradually increased while closely monitoring the baby and mother's contractions. It may feel that Pitocin causes pain, but in reality contractions come on faster than the mother has time to adapt to them, and this is why many women perceive induction to be painful. It is only as painful as a quick labor, which is very painful, of course.

The main risk of induction is induction failure, meaning no progress of labor, and this necessitates a C-section. It is difficult to determine if the C-section takes place because of the induction or because it would have happened anyway. If the baby could not tolerate induced contractions, it would likely not tolerate natural contractions. Also, the labor can stall because of the size or position of the baby, none of which are changed or determined by induction. With that being said, induction that is done too early, before the cervix is ripe, is more likely to fail because exhausted mothers and impatient physicians do not want to proceed with three or four days of induction. Obviously some conditions mentioned above require that the baby is born within a given time, and waiting several days is not an option.

*Please talk about other medications (procedures) for induction used today that you have performed or witnessed.*

There are other induction methods, but the main agent is almost always Pitocin. There is mechanical induction, which consists of stripping the membranes. A similar method consists of a Foley bulb catheter that is placed in the cervix and artificially ruptures the membranes. These methods can sometimes provoke contractions and cervical ripening, and they are routinely used.

*Please talk about pain management and epidural.*

The most popular and effective method to relieve pain with medication is an epidural. Some believe that it may slow down labor. However, as my own experience sometimes showed, it can actually speed up labor when given at the right time. There is no time when it's medically too early or too late to receive an epidural. There is, however, an inconvenient time.

Once an epidural is administered, women are completely immobile and are not in control of their lower extremities. This is uncomfortable because not only are they unable to walk, but they also have to have a bed pan or a catheter placed inside because the bladder becomes too lazy to urinate. Conversely, there is no such thing as too late. But when the delivery is thought to be imminent, it may be that the effect of epidural will not kick in until after the baby is delivered, in which case it will have been an unnecessary procedure. With that being said, the pushing stage can be extremely long for some women (up to three or more hours), and I have seen an epidural placed after one hour of pushing.

The best, most satisfying time when I have seen epidural placed was at about four centimeters, but every labor is different. I have definitely seen it placed at one centimeter and at nine-and-a-half centimeters or even ten centimeters. Also, the epidural is left in place after delivery, which means it is there in case there is extensive repair to be done, or if there is a postpartum bleeding. It seems to me that most women are focused on ten centimeters, and few realize that most of the pain is actually after.

There are, of course, other medication options to consider besides epidural. Stadol, Phenrgan, and Nubaine are often given in the early part of labor in order to deal with painful contractions. These medications often allow the woman to sleep and take the edge off. They are not very effective in active labor, although some women find them helpful. In the very beginning of labor, some women are unable to sleep for several days and are sometimes admitted for rest; they are given Morphine or even Fentanyl to help them sleep. Later in labor these medications can cause respiratory depression in the baby, but in one to two days preceding labor, they can be extremely helpful.

As far as other pain-relief options, there are ways to cope with pain in a non-medicated labor: birthing balls, hot showers, hot tub, squatting bar, and repositioning on hands and knees are some of the methods used when a woman wishes to avoid using medications.

*What do you think a woman should do during pregnancy in preparation for labor and delivery?*

The most important advice I can give is to pick your ob-gyn well. There is no magic formula for this. Just think about it the same way you would pick anyone else who provides you a service, such as a hairdresser, a carpenter, or a contractor. It has to be someone with whom you are comfortable. Your doctor should listen to your needs, answer your questions, and be accessible. Most importantly, your personalities should match! It is important to listen to which doctors your friends liked, and why, but to keep in mind that your needs may be very different from theirs. Doctors have personalities, and while they may be respected and well-known, you may just not like them. You may be better suited for a small community doctor or a midwife who likes to deliver her own patients, and will spend the majority of laboring time with you. On the other hand, you might be very scientifically inclined and need detailed, academic explanations with statistical information. Or maybe you are comfortable with a large group practice and like seeing a variety of doctors during pregnancy.

Open a dialogue and let your doctor know what you want out of this experience and how much explanation you require. Do not assume that the doctor should know your questions. Patients are very different and so are doctors; we are all only human. Do not be afraid to switch if you are not happy, because you have to be with this person for nine months!


*In closing, please share a unique labor experience you have observed during your career?*

It was four in the morning, and I got paged: new patient coming up, second baby, four centimeters, would really like an epidural.

A tiny frightened Guatemalan woman was sitting at the edge of the bed confused by what the anesthesiologist was trying to tell her. I came up to her and took her little hand into mine, while letting her lean into my shoulder. During the short minute between the intense contractions, I asked her in Spanish about medications and allergies and other nuisances she cared little about. With each contraction, her grip would tighten on my arm and a tear would roll from her cheek onto my shoulder, yet she remained quiet. Her calmness was not deceiving me—something about her intensity did not look like four centimeters.

The anesthesiologist just finished placing the catheter. He was ready to inject the medication when suddenly, in complete quietness and composure, she bit me. She actually bit me! I felt tears coming up in my throat. It was a hard bite, followed by a quiet whispering, "That's it."

That's it? Still holding my arm, she leaned to her right, and we all heard a cry. This time it was coming right from underneath her. A baby girl rolled out effortlessly onto the bed.

I guess it wasn't four centimeters after all.

# Interview with a midwife

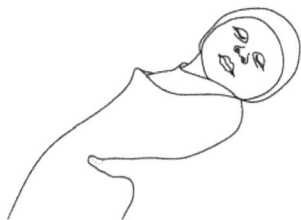

*Debra Ames is a certified nurse midwife at a hospital in Western Massachusetts, who has been practicing since 1984. Debra received her nursing degree from Curry College. She holds a Certificate in Midwifery from University of Mississippi Medical Center and is certified by the American College of Nurse-Midwives. Throughout her career, Debra assisted during two-to-three thousand births. She chose to become a midwife so that she could empower women to make choices about their labor experiences.*

*What is your philosophy about childbirth?*

Childbirth is a natural process, and it is our job as providers to support women's natural, innate strength.

*How do you talk to your patients about pain during childbirth?*

I tell my patients that labor is overwhelming and can be perceived as painful, but the human body is doing the job it is made to do, and there are ways of dealing with pain, such as concentrating on something else, taking baths, or taking medications that may help them relax. I explain to them that the more pain management we introduce, the more we interfere with the natural process. I tell them that each woman has control over how she will manage the experience of pain and ask them how they would like to manage it. I also tell them that being in pain might feel like you're not in control, but really you are. I explain to them that the more accepting they are to labor as a natural process, the easier the labor will be. I describe the breaks in between the contractions as little oases and try to break labor into half-hour slots. I also stress that at the end there will be a baby and a lot of big smiles.

*How powerful have you observed your words to be in helping women get through the pain during labor?*

Language is very powerful. There is a point at which every woman hits the wall and asks for an epidural. What she is really saying is that she feels helpless. I tell them that the pain will go away soon, that I won't leave them, and that we will do this together. At the end, I often hear women tell me, "I am so proud that I did that." I find that preferable to "I couldn't have done that without the epidural."

Epidurals are culturally supported, and it has become the way for American women to give birth, but it is not the only way. Hospitals support epidurals because they keep a quiet area, and they make women easier to manage. Having said that, I'm not against epidurals by any means. My goal is to hear a women say, "I did this, and I chose to do it this way," regardless of whether they chose to have a natural or medicated birth.

*What is your view on induction for pregnancies that go beyond the due date?*

If the woman is past her due date and there are no problems with her tests, there is no need for an induction. I do support inductions for pregnancies that go past forty-two weeks or with any medical indication.

*What is your view on C-sections and what have you seen to be the most common reasons for them?*

C-sections happen too often. A C-section rate of ten to fifteen percent is appropriate in a healthy population, but today's rate is over thirty percent. The most common reason for a C-section is repeat elective C-section. Other common reasons are breech presentation and failure to progress. The C-sections that occur because of failure to progress are often a result of failure to properly understand the normal course of labor and incorrect intervention. The chances of having a C-section depend on numerous things, such as whether you are in a small town or a big city, how people view labor, what kind of medical setting you are in, and the amount of patience for how long a labor can last. Some of these factors can warp the natural experience and hinder the progress of labor to create a scenario that requires a C-section.

*What pharmaceutical drugs, homeopathic medicine, and/or herbs do you use at births?*

I have used Blue Cohosh in late pregnancy to help tone the uterus. Before birth and on the due date, I have used evening primrose oil. This is used inter-vaginally in order to help ripen the cervix. I have also used a narcotic called Stadol and epidural anesthesia.

*What do you consider a high-risk pregnancy?*

A high-risk pregnancy is when the woman has preexisting medical conditions, such as high blood pressure, diabetes, or any other preexisting condition that could adversely affect her pregnancy. I also consider twin pregnancies high-risk, simply because it's harder to gestate two babies. Some other high-risk conditions that arise as a result of pregnancy are placenta previa and intrauterine growth retardation.

Some women will come in and say that they have a high-risk pregnancy. I prefer to say that they have special considerations because these are issues that need attention and consideration. The conditions above would be considered high-risk for a home birth.

*What are the ways in which your job differs between a home and a hospital delivery?*

I do not have much experience assisting at home births. It is a big responsibility because if anything goes wrong, being at home makes it more difficult to take care of the situation. In a home birth, there are not as many interventions. There are no fetal monitors and there are no epidurals. In a hospital, women are monitored and almost universally use pain relief. For the woman, a hospital is never home. At home, no one would enter your space without asking for permission, but in a hospital, people are always in and out of the room. When a woman is at home, there is more respect all around. Having said that, some women will feel more comfortable at home, and others will feel more comfortable at the hospital.

*Please describe some complications that you handled, and how they would apply to a homebirth?*

The most common complication after birth is postpartum hemorrhage. I do a uterine massage and give medication to contract the uterus. Another complication is a baby who is not breathing at birth. One can rarely predict that. In this scenario, you have to resuscitate the baby. If you're attending a home birth, then you must be able to deal with this responsibility. A hospital always has a trained pediatrician. It is important for the woman to understand that she does not have the same resources at home.

*What, in your opinion, has changed the most in the perception of childbirth since you became a midwife?*

Now, people falsely believe that C-sections are easy, and there is growing universal usage of epidurals. Today, women believe it is their right to not feel the pain of childbirth, but they don't always understand the trade-off.

*Why would a woman choose a midwife over an ob-gyn?*

If a woman wants personalized care she should choose a midwife. I am usually there during the early stage of labor, during the active stage, and when the time comes to deliver the baby. When I was in a full practice, I would support everyone the entire night and stay with the laboring woman. However, not all midwives practice in this way.

If a woman chooses a doctor, the doctor will be there if something goes wrong, but he/she is not there supporting her throughout the labor. The nurse will be taking care of her; the doctor will be in and out of the room. There is a lot less attention to the woman in labor. Once she has the epidural, everyone takes a nap.

*Do you think there is a benefit to a doula, and if so, what kind?*

There is definitely a benefit to a doula. Studies have shown that women experience less anxiety and pain in labor with the addition of a doula. Also, if a woman chooses a health-care provider who is not dedicated to be with her in labor, a doula can provide this service. A doula provides additional support and can also be a key communicator between the woman and her midwife or doctor.

I think a woman should interview a doula prior to engaging her services to see if they are a personal and philosophical fit.

*What sources of information do you recommend to women who are preparing for labor?*

I always liked *Birthing from Within* and also recommend any of the books on hypnobirthing. I would also look into childbirth preparation classes that are small in size, as well as some of the classes that are not associated with a hospital.

Women should view birth as a transition from not being a mother to being a mother. It is also important that they try to reduce their fear. Childbirth shouldn't be a scary experience; it should be a powerful one. Sometimes you can reduce fear through knowledge and sometimes through relaxation.

Any woman having a baby should consider all of her options and realize that she has the right to get good care. If you have some choice, you should exercise it. It is of the utmost importance whom you choose to have with you at the birth. Use word of mouth. Go with your gut. Do whatever you need in order to feel comfortable with your choice. If you don't like someone, do you want them to see you naked? You want whomever you choose to advocate for you!

Repose in the pose

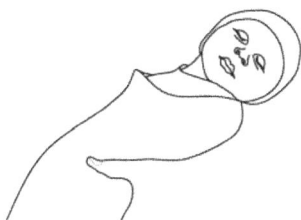

*Catherine is an attorney and a stay-at-home mom who was successful at non-medicated birth. This mother was a gymnast growing up, and has been practicing yoga for a number of years. She took natural birth classes to prepare herself for labor, hired a doula to be a part of her support team, and did research to educate herself on the process of labor and how the body can cope with it.*

*This story is important because while we encourage you to keep an open mind to different types of labor experiences, we are thrilled to share with you an experience where a mother was able to have the exact type of labor that she wanted.*

*What is also very important in this story is to see how correct a mother's instincts can be while she is in labor. This mother was able to recognize each stage in the progression of her labor before anyone else. And while her instincts were not always met with agreement from the hospital staff, she always remained confident in what she was feeling. She was able to listen to her body and knew exactly what was happening to her.*

My husband and I took a Bradley Child Birth Class in preparation for the birth of our baby boy. The class is an extremely in-depth look at the labor process, and it is geared toward non-medicated birth. At Bradley, the husband is viewed as the coach in childbirth. Even though my husband was well-educated, we decided that having a doula would allow him to be relaxed and present for me emotionally.

We interviewed a few doulas, and we really liked the personality of the one we chose. She was the strong motherly type, calm, collected and knew exactly what she was doing. She also clicked with my husband's personality. He liked that he was able to joke with her and be himself. She had extensive experience that included more than three-hundred births, and she was training to become a midwife. She was also a La Leche League leader for many years, so I knew she would be there to give me breastfeeding help right after the birth.

Five days before my due date, I woke up in the early hours of the morning feeling like some liquid escaped. I went to the bathroom to assess the situation and realized that it was a bit of the amnionic fluid. I woke up my husband and told him I thought my water broke. He jumped up half-asleep, totally disoriented and said in a panicked voice, "What do we do now?" I replied, "Nothing else is happening so go back to sleep." He did, and I called my doula, who instructed me to stay close to home, rest, walk, and call her throughout the day to let her know how I was doing. As the day continued, I slept, watched TV, did a lot of walking, ate, and felt some Braxton Hicks contractions, which were painless but frequent. I noticed a bit of mucus and blood discharge as the day progressed, but no more water leakage. As it got closer to nighttime, my doula said she would come over to my house to see if she could help get my contractions going.

She arrived in the evening. At first she was simply keeping me company and providing emotional support. She had a handheld Doppler and was able to check the baby's heartbeat to make sure everything was fine. She asked me to go to bed and brought me a homeopathic remedy to strengthen contractions every fifteen minutes. My contractions started to become stronger after midnight. A few hours later, I came into the living room to sit on a birthing ball. My contractions were about five minutes apart throughout the night, gradually increasing in intensity. As the morning hours approached, each contraction required more and more concentration. I kept laboring through the morning, and my doula was right there to suggest different positions. I was mostly on the birthing ball, and as the contractions increased, I moved onto the rocking chair, which was very relaxing because I did not have to use my muscles. My doula read me a passage from a book that had me focus on different body parts, and it almost put me to sleep. She also massaged some of the pressure points on my shins and around the ankles, and this relieved some of the pain. The biggest help of having her while I was home was that I felt comfortable. I had an experienced woman by my side guiding me. I didn't have to be concerned about anything. I knew that I was in great hands and that everything was fine.

As the day progressed and lunchtime rolled around, my husband went out to get us something to eat. At that point, I could not eat a lot, and I was not getting out of my rocking chair. I did eat some food because it was important for me to keep my energy up. After lunch my labor was definitely a lot harder. My contractions were getting stronger, and my husband and I started walking around the back yard. It was a beautiful day, and we held hands while we walked around. Whenever a contraction came, I leaned on him and breathed through it. By late afternoon my contractions were definitely hard, but still five minutes apart, and I was glad to be at home because I felt relaxed and not rushed. During my labor, I asked my doula when I should go to the hospital, and she said I would know the right time. At one point, she suggested I put my chest on the birthing ball and my knees on the floor. As soon as I did that my contractions changed, and I had three or four contractions that were two minutes apart. I knew it was time to go to the hospital. I asked my doula to check my dilation, and she said I was at six centimeters.

When we arrived at the hospital, we gave the nurses our written birthing plan, of which I brought a number of colored copies. My doctor signed off on all provisions dealing with the birth. Our plan basically stated that I did not want to be continuously monitored or have an IV, and I wanted to have a non-medicated birth without much intrusion. The hospital I chose tries to match like-minded nurses with mothers who want a natural birth. These nurses know how to handle natural birth, how to monitor the baby by hand intermittently, and understand the difference between a medicated and non-medicated birth.

It was good to have my doula in the hospital with me because she was helping us navigate through the hospital bureaucracy. If I was unsure about something, I could turn to her and ask. She also knew the hospital staff, which gave her credibility. After we checked in at the hospital, they asked me if I was in labor. I responded, "Most definitely," somewhat surprised, and they said they would have the staff doctor check me to make sure. If I were not in pain, I would probably think the whole thing was pretty funny. They took me to a room and the doctor checked my dilation and agreed that I was in labor. She also remarked that my water had not broken. While I was laboring at home I was taking a lot of Vitamin C and Echinacea because I thought my water had broken, and I wanted to prevent any infections. My doula said the water probably leaked really high up, but didn't break. I was happy knowing that it didn't break, because if it had, hospital staff would be concerned about the risk of infection and would want to intervene in my labor if it didn't progress within a certain amount of time. I certainly did not want to receive antibiotics during labor.

After the staff doctor checked me, I was left with two wonderful nurses, my doula, my husband, and my mother, who joined me at the hospital. My doula was behind me, and my mom and my husband were on each side. This was my support team. Then the rest of the family arrived: my father, my grandparents, and my husband's family. They walked into the labor room and took some pictures. I still have the photographs of me smiling, which is amazing considering that labor was getting difficult. Soon after that, my contractions became very strong, and my husband asked all of the family members to go into the waiting room, except my birthing team. In my room, I was not hooked up to anything, the voices were kept low, and the room was dark. The only thing I had to concentrate on was each contraction. My doula placed a birthing ball at the corner of the bed, and I sat on it leaning over the bed with my mom exerting light pressure on my lower back with her hands. My mom is a massage therapist, and she was an incredible source of help and support.

My mom, the doula, and my husband traded off giving me juice through a straw. Although we packed a whole cooler of food for the hospital, I didn't have an appetite anymore. I switched to ice chips because that's all I could handle. I also ate some honey because I knew it would give me a quick sugar boost. My only monitoring included about fifteen to twenty minutes to establish a base line of the baby's heartbeat. The unbelievable moment of my labor experience occurred when I was being monitored by my doula, and she told my husband to speak to the baby; every time he spoke the baby's heart rate went up. It was incredible! At first we thought it was a coincidence, but he kept doing it, and the baby's heart beat kept going up. After this initial monitoring period, I was only monitored by hand every thirty minutes through one or two contractions. It was wonderful not having any straps around my belly because I needed room to move.

At some point, when I was laboring at the hospital, my doula suggested I labor on the toilet. I got up, and my husband led me to the toilet. I sat down on it with my husband supporting me, and as the contraction came there was a loud plop. My bag of water had burst. It could not have burst in a more convenient place. I still don't know how my doula knew! After that, it got hard! I got on the bed on my knees, and the doula put the ball on the bed so that I could rest my body over the ball. For some reason, throughout my pregnancy I always knew I would give birth on my hands and knees because that was the position that seemed instinctively comfortable to me. I knew I did not want to be on my back because then I would be working against gravity. Normally when the baby is passing through the birth canal the bones in the lower back expand to allow for the passage of the baby, and my mom actually witnessed that happening to me. As a massage therapist who is acutely aware of the anatomy of the body, she was completely amazed when she saw my bones move. As I assumed my hands-and-knees position over the ball, my mom was on the right, my husband was on the left feeding me ice chips, and my doula was behind me.

My contractions were very strong at that point, and my doula kept reminding me to keep the pitch of my voice low. When I was on my hands and knees, I felt the baby start to descend, and I thought that my doctor should get there as soon as possible. They usually call the doctor at about eight centimeters, and I thought I must be pretty close to that. Before they called my doctor, they wanted to check my dilation. It's funny; the hospital staff does not believe you when you tell them something is happening, so I let them. After checking my dilation they said I was at eight centimeters, my cervix was paper thin, and agreed that it was time to make the call.

By the time my doctor arrived, I was so absorbed in laboring that I don't remember seeing him or whatever else the nurses were doing. I was in my own world, and the only rational thought in my brain was that after each contraction there is a break, and when it gets really difficult that means I'm close to being done. I felt the baby moving down, and I had to push. I had to push as hard as I could. When you're pushing and the head crowns, it's called the ring of fire, and when I felt that, I had to use all my strength and push as hard as I could because that is what my body was telling me to do.

My doctor was wonderful. My husband tells me he just sat in a chair next to my bed and gave quiet instructions to keep the pitch of my voice low. When I felt the baby being born, I said that he was coming. At that point, the doctor was there in a second and ready to catch the baby. I pushed the baby out on my hands and knees. My doctor passed the baby between my legs and laid the baby in front of me. The baby cried. He was red, but looked surprisingly clean, and he had a very strong cry. I kept saying, "Don't cry, don't cry." We waited for about five to ten minutes to clamp his cord until it stopped pulsating—to make sure that he received the proper amount of blood. This is especially important if the baby is slow to start breathing. After a few minutes, I sat up on the bed, and the baby was placed on my chest (skin to skin), and that's when all of us were able to relax and look at one another. That's when the baby stopped crying.

I did not want the first hour of our baby's life to be disturbed, and he nursed for the first time after thirty minutes. After that hour of undisturbed contact, my husband held him for the first time.

The years of yoga I had taken helped me the most during labor. I always tried to keep my body and my face relaxed during the contractions. It allowed me to breathe through each contraction and take it one step at a time. During labor I thought of a phrase my yoga teacher used to say: "Repose in the pose."

He has the drugs; he is my hero

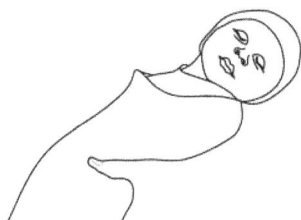

*Denise was a first-time mom, determined to have a non-medicated delivery. She was confident that nothing would stand in her way, spent her time researching natural birth, and assumed breastfeeding would come naturally. She did not consider any other possibilities. But, her labor and delivery did not go as planned.*

*This story takes us through the emotional rollercoaster, as Denise fights with her body and her mind to keep the epidural at bay. We see her lose site of her ultimate goal, the delivery of her baby, and focus entirely on making sure that her baby's birth is non-medicated. Ultimately, though, she gives up on that goal to make sure that her baby is born and that she has the strength to welcome him or her into this world.*

*Denise's labor teaches us that even though in preparation you may have your mind set on things happening a certain way, you do not know how you will truly feel until you are in labor and postpartum. Ultimately, it is okay to change your mind with no guilt and to feel a great sense of accomplishment at the end.*

Going into my birthing experience I was part of the natural camp. There was no way I was going to get an epidural. I had my tonsils taken out without anesthesia; I could handle giving birth without drugs, thank you very much! At a comfortable age of twenty-seven with no major health problems, I was going to pop this baby out in La-La Land, listening to soothing yoga music and looking deep into my husband's eyes. And things were going to get even better after that because my baby would be latched onto my breast round-the-clock as I went about my business, working and keeping up with my fun social schedule. My doctor explained to me that the positioning of the baby necessitated back labor, but this did not seem to stress me out at all. I thought, "He'll turn when the time comes."

I was one day past my due date when I suddenly became nervous that the baby was just too comfortable in there and would never come out. I went to get acupuncture and a massage and, coupled with trying other natural ways to speed up labor, I began to feel a bit sick in my stomach two days later. I also called my doula, who told me to have a glass of red wine, take a bath, and go to sleep.

SLEEP?! No, I was lying in my bed, imagining my beautiful baby, having the butterflies in my stomach the way you do before a big day. No sleeping for me—I wasn't going to miss a minute of this!

I did doze off in the end, and was woken up in the middle of the night by very strong cramps, the kind I take an Advil for when I get my period. I woke up my husband and asked him to go to the other room and sleep there, as there was a chance that I was going to make some noise in our bedroom. The cramps lasted about an hour. They became more and more intense with the pain moving away from both sides of my abdomen and crashing into my lower back each time. I could do nothing but accept that I was headed for back labor. Slowly but surely, heavy contractions moved in, replacing the cramps. These contractions were strong grips that began on my hips, pushing on them, squashing life out of them, and converged on my lower back. From then on, I felt almost nothing around my abdomen—it was all in my back. When the doula arrived, there was only a few seconds of rest between contractions; no need to time them. It was a continuous struggle, and I was working very hard.

My apartment is long and stretched out. This was to my advantage because I could pace. It felt as if I was running, but both my doula and my husband told me I was just pacing. It took long enough for me to walk the length of the apartment and back halfway to the baby room, where I plunged myself into the rocking chair and dozed off for a few seconds of heaven in between the contractions. It seemed like an eternity. I remember the shades being drawn: it was easier to be in the dark. I remember screaming at my husband to turn the soothing music off—it wasn't doing any soothing. I remember my husband and my doula talking about the view from our apartment, and I also remember being upset at hearing that conversation. I remember the honey sticks—my doula brought them and made me suck on them because I couldn't eat or drink anything. I remember the bathtub—the infamous bathtub—the torture that it was for me to lay back in the warm water. It intensified everything that I was feeling, and all I wanted to do was jump out. I had to be in constant motion because it was the only way that I could handle the pain.  At one point I got on my bed and leaned on the headrest, while my doula massaged my back.  Then, I felt the urge to use the bathroom, and the mucus plug came out.  My doula checked me, and she thought I was close to five centimeters.  It had been ten and a half hours of laboring at home, and we decided to go to my doctor's office to get checked.

The drive was a blur, and I could feel each bump on the road.  I remember observing people's scared reactions to my grunts and running around the elevator cabin as if I had a drill up my behind.  Then I was checked by my doctor and the verdict was in: ONE.

I was one centimeter dilated.  I just couldn't believe it.  I was sobbing and screaming, and I realized that I was only at the beginning and already my patience had run out.  You would think I would give up?  No.  Instead, I got dressed, and we came back home, back to the pacing and to the pain.  After twelve hours of back labor I came to my senses.  I could not do this anymore.  There was not going to be a Birthing Center, and there was not going to be a natural birth.  All I could say and think was: "I WANT TO GET AN EPIDURAL!"  With that we were back in the car, but this time I knew relief was in sight.  I could feel it coming.

I was lucky to have a great doula with me.  She knew her way around the hospital, and she quickly got me past the registration point, while my husband was left behind filling out paperwork.  We had pre-registered, but for the Birthing Center, not Labor and Delivery, which is where I was headed.  It also didn't occur to me that getting the injection required an IV and a patient's room, none of which were readily available when I arrived.

After being at the hospital for a grueling forty minutes, all that they managed to do was to undress me and get me into the hospital gown, which exposed my behind.  I was running around the floor screaming and begging my doula and my husband to use all of their negotiation skills to get me that injection as soon as possible.  I even told my doula I was dying, which to my great surprise she totally dismissed.

He has the drugs, he is my hero

I finally received an IV and was connected to the monitor. They also inserted a catheter, which meant that the next time I could use the restroom would be after delivery. Then the anesthesiologist arrived. He had a huge needle on his tray, which normally would have sent me off running, but this time I craved it. I hugged my husband, which helped me get into the right position on the bed. We all waited for the contraction to stop so that he could get the needle in between contractions. "Good luck," I thought. After a few minutes of waiting, he told me to hold my breath and not to move. To this day I don't know how I kept myself still as he administered the CSE (Combined Spinal-Epidural). The feeling was magical—I felt nothing.

The next hour and a half were the best of my twenty-four hour labor experience. I didn't feel anything below my waist, and I was coming in and out of sleep with my husband sitting and napping next to me. My parents, who at that point gathered outside my room, were also resting and were in better spirits as they were no longer hearing my screams. I loved that I could hear my son's heartbeat, and I loved watching my contractions on the monitor. I remember thinking how much better it was to just watch them as opposed to feeling them. My doula also went to take a nap; it was downtime in my camp.

What followed was another disappointment: the pain came back. As the spinal wore off, I kept requesting that they add to the epidural, but it did not seem to work. It was terrible, and I could no longer move around the way I did before. Still, this pain was not as bad as the contractions I experienced before arriving at the hospital. I was shaking a lot from the anesthesia and I was incredibly thirsty. I needed ice cubes because drinking liquids is not allowed for a patient with an IV or an epidural, so my mom came in and fed them to me.

Another anesthesiologist was brought in to see if I needed a different shot because they suspected that the first shot did not go in at the right place. Still, the pain remained, but it was a bit more bearable. He said that he had never seen anyone get this much epidural fluid before.

At last, about twenty-three hours into my labor, I was ready to push. I hated being so drugged up because I could not feel anything in the lower part of my body. It was hard to understand how to push, but somehow I did, and it was such relief. I did not feel the pain of the contractions when I made the effort to push. I felt like I was pushing with my chest, and it was an incredibly strange sensation. I could feel nothing but pressure in the birth canal. My doctor had another delivery in the room next to mine, so she left the pushing to my doula and one of the nurses. I didn't feel a lot of pain, and we were giggling and laughing, and it was a fun atmosphere to be in. This was my favorite part of labor. I could feel that I was close to the finish line. There were a few times when the monitors showed the baby's heart rate drop, so my doula would give me an oxygen mask to use, and it would immediately stabilize. It was very comforting to know how the baby was doing every step of the way.

When his head crowned, my doctor came in. She took a look and gestured to my doula that the baby was huge. I later found out that she also made a scissor sign with her fingers, indicating that she may have to do an episiotomy. And just then, my son decided it was time to be born. He was placed on my chest and decided to go to the bathroom right there and then! What a grateful gesture! I could not help but smile.

My parents and my husband all sat around the bed, passing my son around and marveling at him. He was crying on everyone's lap, and even more so when he was on my breast. I suppose this was a good insight into the future week and a half of breastfeeding. In the meantime, he only really settled down with my mom. She held him and looked at him, and they had a good connection which I enjoyed watching.

And that was it. I spent three nights in the hospital with him—I gave him to the nursery for four hours the first night to get a bit of rest. The rest of the time he was with me. We tried desperately to breastfeed, but there was no luck. He was not latching on but was very hungry. By the end of the third day, he turned yellow and my doctor suggested that I give him formula. During my pregnancy, I had imagined an exclusively breastfed baby, but when I saw how dehydrated he was, I did not think twice and gave him the formula that they had at the hospital. We later switched him to Enfamil, and he drank that all the way up to his one-year birthday.

He has the drugs, he is my hero

I recovered easily and quickly. I was walking around one hour after delivery and got my period back six weeks after. The stitches healed in a week, and I did not feel any pain whatsoever in about four weeks. For about ten days after delivery, I would wake up and my bed sheets would be soaking wet. My body was giving up a lot of water.

For about a week-and-a-half the baby and I were miserable. We were trying to breastfeed while supplementing with formula, but I quickly realized that it would not work. To my surprise, even pumping did not happen for me because I would be in too much pain and would give up. The most frustrating thing in those days was that I felt there was no authority to guide me through postpartum. While I loved my doctor and my doula, they really did not concentrate on us too much after the baby was out. We did not like our pediatrician, and did not find one that we liked until my son's third month.

Being a bit depressed, recovering from delivery, and being unable to breastfeed, I wished for a postpartum doula, which was something I actually looked into. If I ever had to be a first-time mother again, I would hire a postpartum doula—the baby will come out one way or the other. It's what to do with him afterwards that really matters.

I admit that I spent too much time preparing for labor during my pregnancy. It was twenty-four hours out of my life that I spent nine months researching, thinking about, and preparing for, but I was not ready for what came next. My husband shared the same sentiments with me. He also felt unprepared for how to deal with the baby's needs. I was not ready for the screaming and crying, for the lack of sleep, for not being able to be a super-mom, and, ultimately, for being totally fine with that. Who was I kidding? As much as I would love to be, I am not in the natural camp, and never will be. I've got a business to run, fun to have, and a life to live. I hired a nanny and went back to being myself. And as for my son, we love each other. He is beautiful, and I am so happy to have him. He says "Mama!" to me in the morning, and for that I forgive the fact that it is 6 a.m. and about two hours earlier than what I would normally call morning.

After things settled down a bit, my husband shared with me that what helped him throughout my pregnancy and labor was being aware of all the hormonal changes that were happening in my body. On the day of labor he remembered that even though he was sorting through a number of emotions, he knew this day was about me and tried to remain in the background and pay attention to my needs. He told me that although he felt powerless seeing me in so much pain, he was proud to watch me proceed with labor in an admirable fashion.

I'm sorry, it's a little girl

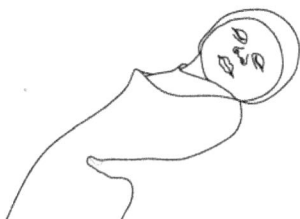

*Because they were a nurse and a doctor, both Diana and her husband were well-versed in the physiological progression of labor and did not feel the need for either a doula or any other support during labor.*

*When Diana was faced with unexpected situations, she did not panic but calmly followed the guidance provided by the medical professionals because they were carefully selected, and she trusted them.*

*However, Diana's story shows that even when you have confidence in your abilities to cope with pain and you are familiar with the labor process, it is still difficult to prepare for the emotions associated with the birth of a child for both the father and the mother.*

I was past my due date, and our doctor recommended that we wait a week before deciding whether to have an induction. My doctor encouraged me to have an idea about how I wanted things to happen, but also said that anything can happen, and we must remain flexible. Since I never went into labor on my own, a week later we went to the hospital. I was immediately connected to an IV, and shortly after that induced with Pitocin. My contractions started about six hours after our arrival at the hospital. Even though I was in active labor, I did not dilate fast enough and was only three centimeters by late evening.

Throughout my labor, my husband was my main source of support. He would say, "Honey, why don't we get some of that lavender lotion, and I'll rub your hands with it? Can I rub your back?" He tried to comfort me by using everything that he learned in birthing classes, but it wasn't helping. I kept saying, "Whatever. Nothing is going to help me now."

I did not consider getting a doula because my husband is a physician. He understood everything and was not nervous about the process, so I did not feel the need to have another person in the room. He knew the residents that were checking on me every hour. Aside from my husband, the nurses were also very helpful.

I got the epidural late in the evening, and I did not feel any pain. After that, I was the happiest girl and went to sleep! The nurses checked my progress every hour. Finally, when I was six centimeters dilated they noticed meconium and decided to break my water. In case of an emergency, two nurses from the Neonatal Intensive Care Unit were present at my delivery. After a few hours of laboring, they noticed that the baby's heart rate was decreasing. A wire was placed on the baby's scalp to do some internal monitoring. A couple minutes later the heart rate went up. Later, the heart rate went down again, and the doctor suggested that we might need to do an emergency C-section if the heart rate continued to slow down. I was asked to stay on my left side so that the baby could get as much oxygen as possible. They even had an oxygen mask for me.

By mid-morning I was fully dilated. I was told to labor down; in other words, they wanted the baby to drop to the lowest position possible, so that I wouldn't have to push for long. I labored down for about an hour, and I began to push after that. It took about forty-five minutes with not that many pushes in between. During the pushing stage, I actually said that I had not worked out for three months and that this was the best work out I had experienced in a long time. My husband was laughing. It went really well! During this stage, they had me in different positions. First I used a birthing bar. The bar was attached to the bed, and they had me lean on it. Next, I laid on my side for a while holding my right leg up. I think this position actually helped progress labor. They let the epidural wear off a little, so I could feel some of the contractions when I started pushing, and I ended up giving birth on my back.

During the pushing stage my husband was by my side, but he was also looking down. We did not know the gender of our baby, so when she came out, he was so nervous that he mistook the umbilical cord for something else and said, "Oh, it's a little boy." The doctor jokingly replied, "I'm sorry, it's a little girl." Even though my husband is a doctor, he almost fainted when he saw the baby's head crown. Later he shared with me that it feels different when it's your baby being born. They suctioned the baby and took her to make sure she was okay and then put her on my tummy.

I think not knowing the gender of our baby helped me focus because I wanted to reach my goal and find out. Later on that day I said, "Honey, I will have another baby in a second."

He was so shocked! The euphoria after birth made me instantly forget the pain I just went though.

After two hours, I passed a huge blood clot. I needed Pitocin again to make my uterus contract, and I also needed a massage of my uterus, which was extremely painful. I was given narcotics so that I could relax again. They explained that sometimes blood clots happen and that there was no reason to worry.

At first, I had a hard time breastfeeding because even though my daughter latched on, it was not a proper latch. My nipples were bleeding, and I started using a nipple shield, which actually forced her to open her mouth wider, and things got better. After a couple of weeks I took off the nipple shield. She was a great eater. I started pumping two weeks before I went back to work and pumped twice a day. I nursed my daughter for six months.

Am I the only one giving birth here?

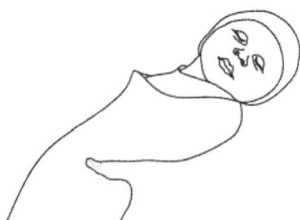

*Emma, a financial analyst and a stay-at-home mom placed her trust in her doctor and agreed to an induction. Unfortunately it was not the right time for the baby to come out, her labor did not progress as expected, and Emma needed a C-section.*

*Even though the surgery was successful and the baby was born healthy, having a C-section took a toll on Emma. She attributes her difficulty in breastfeeding to not being able to get the lactation support she needed when her baby was not latching on properly. Emma was not able to move around much, and as a result, she could not attend breastfeeding classes. Nevertheless, she chose to pump and was able to feed her baby breast milk through a bottle.*

At the end of my pregnancy my doctor and I chose to have a scheduled induction. The reason was that I had a low lying placenta, and also during one of the last appointments the doctor suspected I was going to have a large baby. On the day of the scheduled induction, the baby had not descended, I was not dilated, and my cervix had not effaced yet. A nurse connected me to the monitors so that the hospital staff could track my contractions and my blood pressure.

By evening, I began to feel mild contractions. I also began to dilate, but slowly, only about two centimeters. The decision was made to help me progress by adding Pitocin. After this, I began to have much stronger contractions—they were definitely uncomfortable but still bearable.

In the middle of the night I felt an urge to use the restroom. I noticed blood and called in a nurse to ask her what was happening. I suspected that my water broke, and when the nurse arrived she confirmed that. At this point I was four centimeters dilated and the nurse asked me if I wanted to have an epidural; if so, if I could wait about thirty minutes to get one. I did ask if she thought there was any advantage to waiting, and the nurse did not think there was. I was ready not to have the pain anymore, so I did request an epidural at that time.

By the time the anesthesiologist arrived, my contractions were about one minute apart, so it was very difficult to stay still for the needle, but he did manage to do it in between my contractions. The pain eased almost right away. It felt as though it was a miracle! I could only feel the top of my contractions.

By morning I was still only four centimeters dilated. When the nurse came in to check me, she noted that the baby was in distress. She adjusted the monitors and called my doctor. The doctor's suggestion was to wait for another hour and monitor to make sure the baby was not becoming more distressed.

About an hour later, I was taken off Pitocin because I was only four centimeters dilated and told I was going to have a C-section. I was taken into the operating room and given stronger drugs. I remember shaking, and I was told it was a side effect of the drugs. My doctor was not arriving, and I was informed that another doctor would be doing my surgery, but fortunately my doctor did make it in time. There was a white sheet placed between my head and the rest of my body so I could not see below my chest area. During the surgery I felt some pressure around my belly but not much else. When it was time to take the baby out, my doctor urged my husband to come around the blanket and see the process. My husband agreed. In the next few minutes my baby was born and was given to me to hold for a few minutes before any of the tests. I cried when I held him. I was so happy.

I wanted to breastfeed my baby, and I consulted with the nurses several times during my stay at the hospital about how to nurse. I also found a lactation consultant who helped me with the latch. Unfortunately the latch was a big problem, and it was not working out. It was suggested that I try to pump and that I was able to do. The milk came in and I had a good supply. For the next six months I was able to feed my baby breast milk by using the pump.

I think I might have been able to nurse my baby but the fact that I had a C-section delivery made it more complicated. My recovery was long, and I was not able to go to breastfeeding classes and get adequate help with nursing. I think breastfeeding is very difficult, and although I did prepare for it during my pregnancy by reading breastfeeding books, I was still not able to do it. However, I am happy and proud that my baby did eat breast milk even though it came from a bottle.

When I look back at my labor experience, I have positive memories. The nurses were always coming to check on me, and I felt like I was the only person giving birth there. My husband was a great source of support. It was wonderful having someone to talk to. I couldn't move much, so it was great to have him there next to me because he could help me get places.

We had to put your wife to sleep

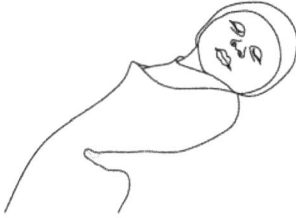

*Isabel, a first-time mother and a business professional, wishes she had prepared differently for the birth of her child. Even though Isabel took a Lamaze class, she thinks the class did not offer enough education about the various options women have today. For instance, she was not aware that she could have had another person, such as a doula, in the delivery room advocating for her. Isabel also wishes she would have had a stronger relationship with her doctor, who would have guided her better, but instead she had to switch doctors three times during her pregnancy.*

*On the upside, not having a written birth plan helped Isabel cope with the way her labor progressed, because it let her accept things as they came. She gave birth to her baby in a way that was possible for her under the circumstances and then had a positive breastfeeding experience.*

When I was about four months pregnant, my doctor announced his retirement. As a result, I visited another associate in the practice for my subsequent appointments. However, by the time I went into labor, the associate I was seeing was due for a vacation. When it was time for me to go into labor, it was yet another doctor who would deliver my child.

Toward the end of my pregnancy, I was put on bed rest for high blood pressure. One day, as I was reading in bed, I felt some contractions. My husband was at work, and I called him to let him know what was happening. He got home early in the evening; my brother and my sister-in-law came over to have dinner with us. The contractions were getting stronger, but I was trying not to make a big deal out of it. We went to bed and kept timing the contractions. They were about five minutes apart, but not very strong. Right before we called the doctor, I felt like I was leaking.

When we arrived at the hospital it turned out my water was indeed leaking, and I was admitted. I was given a sleeping pill so that I could rest. In the morning my contractions were a lot stronger, and the staff administered Pitocin to speed things up.

My husband stepped out for breakfast after I was started on Pitocin. Shortly after he left, several doctors walked into my room and pointed out that they observed something on the monitor. I felt that they were rude and did not explain to me properly what was happening. Unfortunately my husband was not there to help me ask the right questions. All of a sudden, everyone left the room only to come back rushing in ten minutes later. One of the doctors explained that there was something wrong with my baby's heartbeat. I was thrown onto the stretcher and taken into an operating room for an emergency C-section. I was put to sleep in a matter of minutes.

The next thing I remember is my husband, my parents, and my friends at my side. I had no idea what was going on. After I came out of it a little bit, my husband told me we had a baby, and she was in intensive care. I was wheeled into the postpartum room, but on the way we stopped by the intensive care unit so that I could see my baby.

Later I found out that when the baby began to descend, the umbilical cord got tighter around her neck and was wrapped around it twice. My husband also told me that when he came back with breakfast to the maternity wing, the nurses ran up to him and asked if his name was Peter. They said, "We had to put your wife to sleep." They made him wait in a tiny room with no windows. No one came in to explain anything to him until our baby was born. After the immediate danger passed, the doctor did explain to my husband that they had to resuscitate her and that she was having problems breathing. Later in the evening, I saw my daughter. I tried to nurse her, but nothing was happening. She stayed in the intensive care unit for two days. My husband took the video camera and filmed videos of her for me to watch.

During the five days that I was in the hospital recovering, my daughter had formula in the intensive care unit, and then on the third day she began to nurse when she was with me. I did not have any problems with breastfeeding.

The nurses and hospital staff were really great with making sure that I was recovering well. They did a very good job taking care of me and my baby; I was very happy with them. I do not blame the doctor for what happened because when I first got to the hospital, an ultrasound was done and there were no apparent problems. I think the cord wrapped tighter around my baby's neck as the labor progressed. However, I do think there was a lack of communication with my doctor during my pregnancy because my practitioners kept changing. I feel that I might have been more prepared for possible situations if I had more communication with my doctor prior to giving birth and knew more about how my baby was positioned. But I do not regret not having a written plan—I knew that things could go wrong, so I am glad that I did not set myself up for any specific course of events.

Looking back I also feel that I could have prepared differently. I did take a Lamaze class during my pregnancy, but I feel like I was not given adequate information there. For example, I had no idea that it was okay to have a labor without an epidural. Some time later, I went to another Lamaze class with my pregnant friend and learned more about other options. Although I am happy that other women are given many more choices now, I feel I was disadvantaged because of not knowing enough. I also did not hire a doula when I was pregnant because I did not know that this type of support in labor even existed. I am not sure if anything would have gone differently, but I do think I might have been served better by having someone by my side with more experience who could have done a better job explaining to me what was happening.

# At home and at peace

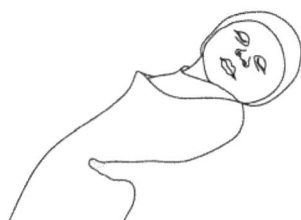

*This first-time mother always wanted to have a non-medicated birth. She discovered that there were no birthing centers where she lived; thus, she decided to have a home birth, which was legal in her state. She felt she was in good health and, after determining that her pregnancy was low-risk, Marilyn did not think she was putting herself in danger by choosing this option. Marylin took the experience of a home birth very seriously and did everything in her power to make it a success by preparing for the big day.*

*This story portrays a mother who was well-trained for a home birth. She took care of herself during her pregnancy and attended a support group for women who have given, or planned to give, birth at home. This helped her learn about the kind of birthing experience she was about to have. She also had full confidence in her support team, and that team proved to be a very good choice. Marylin shows us that if there is trust, and if everyone is on the same page, it is likely to result in a positive outcome.*

I always knew I wanted to have a natural birth, and when I found out there were no birthing centers in the area where I was to give birth, I looked into the option of a home birth. I met with a midwife that I immediately felt comfortable with, and she agreed to be my primary caregiver for the remainder of my pregnancy. She organized regular support groups for her clients (both present and former), and these women were a great resource in preparation for the birth.

Apart from morning sickness during my first trimester, I had a smooth pregnancy. I exercised regularly, ate well, and avoided stressful situations during these nine months.

Four days after my due date, I was out having dinner with my sister and my husband. In an effort to induce labor, I had a glass of wine and some spicy food, both rumored to help get the labor started.

That night, after only two hours of sleep, the contractions began. They came on strong: three to five minutes apart, lasting forty-five seconds on average. In the early hours, I was able to endure the contractions on my own, but in the morning I called our midwife to inform her of my labor. She came over to the house about an hour later, and then two support midwives showed up shortly thereafter.

By the time the other two midwives arrived, I was already oblivious to my surroundings. I felt the contractions acutely in my lower back and was most comfortable when someone was applying pressure to that area. It was great having the support of my husband and three midwives, as someone was always available to assist me with my needs. I changed positions often between the shower, a birthing ball, and a glider ottoman. When my midwife informed me that I was six centimeters dilated, I asked if there was anything she could do to speed up the process. She advised me to walk up and down the stairs with my husband as my support. We followed her advice and tried to do the walking in between contractions. Doing this did progress my labor.

The transition phase was the most difficult stage for me. It felt like I was having contractions and feeling the urge to push simultaneously. At this point, my body felt as if it wasn't sure what to do. Once the pushing phase started, I was able to enjoy the time in between the pushes. I was lying on the bed holding my husband's hands; he was sitting behind me as my support, while the midwives were at the other end of the bed supporting my legs and stretching them out in between the pushes.

Just a few pushes from the actual birth, I felt ready to give up on the labor because I was so exhausted. However, with some encouragement from my husband and midwives, I was able to gather up the needed energy for the final minutes of pushing.

My baby was born shortly thereafter with a nine out of ten rating on the Apgar scale. My labor had lasted a total of nine and a half hours.

I didn't have any problems nursing, and he was exclusively breastfed. Overall, I had a very positive labor experience. Giving birth to my son in the comfort of our home prevented any anxiety associated with the trip to the hospital and any unknowns we may have encountered there. I had complete confidence in my team of midwives who regularly monitored both my health as well as my baby's. I felt relaxed throughout the labor and knew that I was getting the same, if not better, care that I would have received in the hospital. Most of all, I am thankful for having had this opportunity to bring my baby into such a welcoming and comfortable environment.

I willed her to breathe

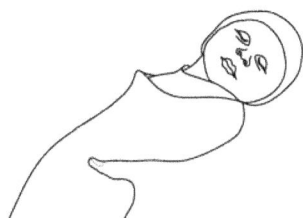

*Ann is a first-time mother and a business owner who had to face a complication after her delivery. Her daughter was born premature and, as a result, her lungs did not fully develop.*

*Ann's story teaches us that although there may be complications, it is possible to overcome them with strength and perseverance. Ann shares with us how unprepared she was for the possibility that something may go wrong. She also shares with us her fears and doubts about her ability to take care of a newborn on her own.*

*This story takes us through many unexpected moments that first-time mothers often face. Although Ann knew that her water may break, she did not know the signs to watch out for to determine if the water breaking might be an indication that the baby is in distress. And, although she took the time to pre-register at the hospital where she would be delivering, she did not realize that more paperwork would be needed upon her arrival during labor.*

About three weeks before my due date, I woke up in the middle of the night to go to the bathroom. I felt a bit of cramping but attributed it to having eaten something. After using the bathroom, I was still uncomfortable—something was hurting. I used the bathroom a couple more times, and on the third time, I managed to jump out of bed before my water broke. When I realized the cramps I was feeling were contractions, I began to time them. They were five to ten minutes apart.

My doctor did not discuss with me that when water breaks it should be clear. Mine was not, and I did not know that my baby was in distress. I was not worried about the contractions because during the last trimester of my pregnancy I experienced a lot of painful Braxton Hicks contractions, and I was used to the pain.

I decided to go to the hospital because I remembered that my mother birthed both of her children very quickly, and I wanted to be near the hospital in case my labor was also fast.

The drive to the hospital was not long. It was the middle of the night, so there was a lot less traffic than usual. When we arrived at the hospital, I noted what a beautiful, state-of-the art medical facility I was in. We chose to pre-register at this hospital because we'd heard wonderful reviews about it and because my doctor was an attending doctor there.

What I did not realize was that even though we pre-registered at the hospital, there was still some paperwork that we had to fill out upon our arrival. My water was leaking, and I was in a great deal of pain. I was also paranoid that I would not make it in time to have an epidural, as I thought that there was a point when it would be too late to administer it. I was so frustrated that I began to cry. I felt slightly better after the IV was put in, and I received more fluids. Seeing my parents also made me very happy. My support team was now in place.

When my doctor arrived and examined me, I was about six centimeters dilated. I was in a lot of pain, and I was crying. All I could think was that I would be fine once I got the epidural. The anesthesiologist was saying something to me, but I could not understand him. I held my mom by one hand, and my doctor by the other. The drugs began to work instantly, and it was wonderful. I took an hour-long nap while my husband sat by my side. My parents and other family members, who were gathering in the hospital, waited in the hall.

When I woke up I was a bit uncomfortable—I have no tolerance for pain—so I was given a bit more epidural. At that point I was also fully dilated, so it was time to push. My daughter was born after only twenty minutes of pushing. My doctor needed to perform an episiotomy. We discussed this possibility ahead of time, and I was comfortable with having this procedure done if my doctor felt it was needed.

When my daughter was born, she looked exactly like my husband. After she came out, she was taken to another room in order to perform tests and to clear out her lungs. I do not remember her crying. She was perfect: scored well on the tests and did not swallow any meconium. After being cleaned and wrapped into a receiving blanket, she was given to me to hold.

After labor and delivery, I was taken to a private room. I tried to breastfeed, but I worried about staying with my daughter alone overnight. I wanted to make sure someone watched her and I was worried that I may fall asleep. I asked the staff to take my daughter into the nursery and instructed them to bring her to me as soon as she cried.

In the morning I was well-rested and was feeling well. I planned on taking my daughter to a hospital class to learn about feeding her and taking care of her. I was concerned about breastfeeding. While my doctor told me that colostrum was enough for a two-to-three-day old baby, the nurses at the hospital were telling me that she was not eating enough and that she may need formula. I stuck with my doctor's advice, but, of course, I was nervous. I felt that nursing was not going well because my daughter was not latching on properly. She was small, and I thought my nipples were not brought out enough. Prior to giving birth, I assumed that breastfeeding would be easy, but I was finding out that it was not. The class we took was helpful. Among other tips, I was shown how to give her milk through a straw to avoid nipple confusion. We tried it and it worked, so I was less worried about how much milk she was getting.

I thought of taking my daughter to another feeding class, but first I wanted to change her diaper. When we reached the room, I suddenly realized that she turned blue. Panicked, I ran back to the class I had just taken and showed my daughter to the teacher. She picked her up and woke her. She began to breathe again. Quickly, my daughter was taken to the nursery, connected to monitors, and put under a heat lamp. I thought I was losing my baby.

By the time my husband arrived, she was taken to the neonatal intensive care unit (NICU). The doctors were performing tests to see what was wrong. I suspected that something was wrong with her heart because my husband had a heart problem when he was born and even had to have surgery for that later on during his childhood.

The doctors explained to me that because my daughter was born premature, her lungs were slightly undeveloped. This caused her breathing to slow down sometimes if she went into a very deep sleep. She was kept in the NICU for a week until she was stronger, and she was given antibiotics and fluids. She also had a pulse monitor attached to her finger and was given oxygen while in the incubator. I had to take her out to breastfeed, but feedings were very tough, as she was not latching on. As a result,

I had to pump, store the milk, and give it to her from a bottle. I stayed in the hospital most of the time, and so did my mom. My husband stayed one night but needed to return to work after that. To this day, I still think that I willed her to breathe and come back to life.

When we arrived home, the first few nights were very difficult. I was terrified. I brought this little baby home and felt like I should be giving her attention, but I did not really know how. I was constantly scared of her breathing. I woke up with her, fed her with pumped milk, changed her, put her to bed, and then pumped again. This was my routine. I would be up for two hours pumping and had about an hour of sleep until she woke up again.

Luckily, I had a lot of help from my family. Although my husband needed to work, my grandmother came every day for the first two weeks after we returned from the hospital. Later, she continued to come and help me two to three times per week for the first year of my baby's life.

It isn't easy, even the second time around

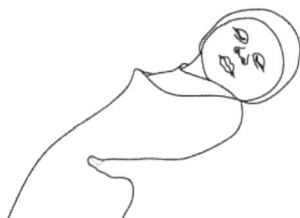

*Jane had already birthed one child and was not able to breastfeed him. She spent a lot of time and effort preparing to breastfeed her second child. After almost two months of hard work at breastfeeding, she and her family made the choice to switch to formula, because they felt the experience was not working for the baby as well as for the family as a whole.*

*As you read this story, keep in mind that just because in the end it did not work out for this family, it does not mean that you will not be able to turn their experience into a success story. The important task is to understand what went wrong and to learn about what you may do, should you be faced with similar problems of your own.*

Two months before my due date, my doctor told me he planned to go fishing with his son and that he will be out of town around the time my baby was due. I was worried that some strange doctor was going to deliver my baby. Fortunately, things didn't exactly go that way, and our baby arrived earlier than expected.

It all began late in the morning. I was feeling very light cramps, but I had my doubts about it being the real thing because I saw my doctor the day before, and he told me that my cervix had softened, but I was only one centimeter dilated; he asked me to make an appointment in a few days. That night, we had plans to go out with friends to an Art Museum for a Latin party, so mentally I wasn't ready to go into labor just yet. I had made arrangements with my parents for my older son to spend the night at their house that evening so I knew that if anything were to happen, he would be taken care of.

I managed to sleep for a couple of hours and eventually woke up because the cramps were getting stronger, but still very bearable. These contractions were only twenty minutes apart, progressing to fifteen minutes apart in the next couple of hours. I was feeling well, and we decided to go out because we thought it would be better to be out with people, walking around, looking at paintings, and listening to music instead of focusing on the pain.

We met our friends and spent about two hours at the museum. Meanwhile I was timing my contractions. They were about ten minutes apart, but I was still okay. On our way back to the car, I had to stop during my contractions because they were starting to get painful. However, I was pretty hungry and thought I could probably handle another hour of being out. We went to a restaurant, and I ordered a light salad. At one point during dinner, everything became a bit blurry, and I began to tune out from the pain. It finally hit me: "I am in labor." We were nowhere near the hospital, which would have been better for my peace of mind. I interrupted my friend, turned to my husband and said, "We need to go now." "Well, here we go again," my husband replied. He later told me that at this moment he was mentally prepared for what was coming, because he was already there for me once before when our first son was born. By the time we arrived home, my contractions were five to seven minutes apart. We tried walking around the house, but the pain seemed to get worse and worse. Every time I felt a contraction I would just stop and try to breathe through it. Then I decided that I would lie down and try to get some sleep, but I was not able to sleep through such painful contractions. I actually purchased a birthing ball that day, but it was not really helping me to deal with the pain. I was absolutely miserable, but I still held myself together. In fact, what I found the most helpful was to just lean back on the couch, slide to the edge, and spread my legs during the contractions.

When I called my doctor, I was in for a little surprise. I told him that my contractions were five to seven minutes apart and that I was planning to go to the hospital. You can imagine the expression on my face when he named a hospital I had never heard of and told me to wait a little longer. I said, "Do you mean St. Luke's?" and he said, "No, St. Joseph's. I am here until 6 a.m., so if you want me to deliver the baby, you better head over here. If you go to St. Luke's, my partner will have to do the delivery if you deliver before 6 a.m. I won't have enough time to drive over there." All of a sudden I became stressed! We debated for about an hour whether we should go or wait. I went to the bathroom to wash my face and yelled, "Time!" which was my way of telling my husband to time the contractions. When we realized that I was contracting every two minutes, we made the decision to get going.

My husband helped me walk to the emergency room and the lady who greeted us asked me to sit down so she could register me (I had pre-registered, but now I was being admitted to a different hospital, so I had to go through the entire process again). She asked, "What is your name? What is your address? What is your social security number?" She was nice enough to pause during my contractions. Finally, the last question was, "What is your religion?" At that moment I thought to myself, "Is that in case I die during labor?" It took twenty minutes to get registered, and then someone came down, put me in a wheelchair, and took me to the delivery suites.

Once we rolled into the room, I was disappointed. The room wasn't as nice as the one in the hospital where I had planned to deliver, so I started to doubt whether the quality of care would be the same. As soon as I got up from the wheelchair, I felt another painful contraction. The nurse told me to stand up, put my elbows on the bed, and to lean forward. I found that helpful. She gave me a gown and asked me to lie down. My husband was by my side the entire time. He was calm and collected. He later told me that he was proud of me and that he was thankful for how strong and prepared I was. Shortly after that, another nurse walked in and hooked me up to a monitor and an IV. I thought about asking them not to do that, but my contractions were getting more painful, and I remembered that during my first labor I preferred to either sit or lie in bed. I had also planned on getting an epidural, and I knew that I had to be hooked up to the IV in order to get it. I didn't think it would be wise to postpone the inevitable. When the nurse told me that I would be able to get my epidural shortly I panicked a little and told her that I did not want it until I was five centimeters dilated. I was afraid of slowing down my labor, so she checked. You can imagine how happy I was when she told me that I was at five and that I could be free of pain. At one point my doctor walked in to check on me; he explained that he would be resting down the hall and would check on me from time to time. Next, the anesthesiologist walked in. One of the first questions he asked me was to describe any previous experiences I may have had with epidurals. I told him that during my previous labor the anesthesiologist missed the first time. He explained to me that anyone can miss, and there are no guarantees. He was very upfront with me and explained the entire procedure in great detail. He told me to sit on the edge of the bed and to arch my back and shoulders, and began his work. He also told me how long it would take to dull the pain and to call him if I still felt painful contractions in fifteen to twenty minutes. Since the pain remained pretty strong I did end up calling him back. In fact, I had to call him back twice because even though I did not experience as much pain as I did before, I pretty much felt all the contractions on the left side.

The nurse was in the room most of the time, and she was absolutely amazing. I felt that I could trust her, and she stayed by my side when my husband needed to leave the room. When the anesthesiologist came back, he told me that sometimes the anesthesia is not distributed evenly. I noticed the look on my husband's face; I could see how disappointed he was that I may need to continue to be in pain. The anesthesiologist also said that he can take out the catheter and start over to see if he can remove all the pain, but again, there were no guarantees. I asked the nurse to check me again, and she said that I was eight centimeters dilated. When I heard that, I realized that the end was in sight, and I chose to manage the pain on one side rather than risk being in pain on both sides.

Some time went by, I had some more strong contractions, and my husband always remained by my side. My doctor walked in to check if I was fully dilated and said that I was at ten centimeters. All of a sudden a few nurses stormed into the room with equipment. One of them stood on one side and my husband was on my other side, and I was screaming like a crazy lady. They were telling me to push, and I was just screaming and screaming. Then I heard, "Jane, Jane, Jane." The doctor was trying to get my attention: "Jane, the baby is not going to come out if you keep screaming. You need to inhale, hold your breath, and push. You've done this before." So, I tried to push as hard as I could. At one point I remember the nurse yelling, "Dad, hold her leg up." I screamed, "That's it. I'm done. I'm not pushing anymore. I've had enough. This hurts! Ahhhh!" Later my husband told me that it was the most surprising moment for him during the entire labor; he could not believe that I said I would not push anymore!

I actually felt the baby's head crown, and it was the most excruciating pain I had ever felt. Once the head was out, the rest of his body was not as bad. The pushing stage lasted fifteen minutes; everything happened very fast. The doctor did make an incision, and because this time my epidural did not fully work, I did feel some pain when he was stitching me up. He gave me a local anesthetic and the procedure took only a few minutes. About four hours went by from the time we arrived at the hospital until delivery.

When David was born, the doctor asked my husband if he wanted to cut the umbilical cord, and he declined. The doctor cut the cord and handed the baby to me. I held my most adorable baby for a little bit and then gave him to the nurses so they could weigh him, measure him, and perform the Apgar test. Since I delivered early in the morning, the lactation consultant was not there yet and one of the nurses told me to latch the baby on as soon as possible.

Even though I considered putting together a birth plan, I decided that it would be best to talk to the nurses and tell them what I wanted instead of handing them a piece of paper. I think it was the right decision because even during my contractions I was still able to voice my concerns.

My most negative memory was the sudden change of plans about where I would deliver the baby. When I found out I would have to go to a different hospital, I was already in a lot of pain and the extra stress of where to go was upsetting to both my husband and me.

Even though things did not go exactly like I had wanted them to, everything worked out for the best. The nurses were caring, sympathetic and took great care of me. I felt that people wanted the best for our family. They always informed me before they did anything and asked for my permission. Both my husband and I were very happy that I delivered David at this hospital.

\*     \*     \*

My first breastfeeding experience helped me realize that breastfeeding was not as natural as I thought, so I decided to prepare seriously for nursing my second baby. I read several books and attended La Leche League meetings prior to his birth. Even though the books I read addressed various potential problems, they made me think that I should be able to breastfeed no matter what. A common theme throughout the books was: If you have breasts, you should be able to breastfeed. At one of the meetings, I met a woman who was unable to nurse her first baby but was successful with the second one. Meeting her was very empowering, and it gave me confidence in myself. I did not let myself have any doubts about my ability to breastfeed because that would minimize the chance of success. I refused to accept the possibility that it may not work out. Unlike my first pregnancy, when I thought breastfeeding was natural and everyone could do it, I was well prepared this time.

At the hospital, one of the questions I was asked was, "Are you going to nurse, or should we give the baby formula?" Without any hesitation, I replied that I was definitely going to nurse my baby and even asked the nurse not to give him a pacifier in order to avoid nipple confusion. I also requested immediate assistance with nursing right after the birth.

After David was born, the nurse who came to help me took my breast and the baby's head and tried to bring him to my nipple. At that time, David wasn't really interested in the breast and wanted to sleep. We tried undressing him and putting a wet cloth on his face, but he was just not interested. The nurse suggested that we try to use a nipple shield, which helped him latch on. However, when the lactation consultant arrived, she was very disappointed and told me to stop using the shield because I would have problems later on. After about fifteen minutes of struggling without using the nipple shield, we did manage to latch him again. At the suggestion of my husband, who thought it was very important that I learned to do this on my own, I tried to latch David on by myself at the next feeding; when I could not do it, I had to call in a nurse to help me. The entire time I was in the hospital, I had someone assisting me at every feeding, and I thought things were going well because he was nursing. The lactation consultant was even able to latch him on after the circumcision, and apparently that was a good sign. When I left the hospital, I knew exactly what to expect, and I thought I was well prepared for the future. According to the lactation consultant, if I could make it through the next three to five days of the engorgement, it would be smooth sailing after that.

During my first day home I had problems latching him on, but I somehow managed. However, during the first night home, David screamed for one and a half hours because my husband and I just could not latch him on, and I refused to use the nipple shield. Finally, he was so tired that he just fell asleep. At six in the morning, we rushed to the hospital. The lactation consultant had not come to work yet, and an older, experienced nurse was called to help me. The baby was screaming. She suggested I use the breast pump to pull out the nipple and to see if some milk will come out. A little bit did come out, and finally, she managed to latch him on. The nurse noticed that my breast was red, and she explained that I should take hot showers before feedings and massage it with baby oil to help get the milk to flow in the milk ducts. As the day continued, the situation did not improve. The pumping and the showering didn't help very much. The only way I could get him to latch on was by using the nipple shield; I had to feed him somehow.

The next day, my right breast was red and enormous, and I didn't know what to do. I had heard that cabbage leaves are helpful in these types of situations, so I just kept putting cold cabbage leaves on my breasts to alleviate the pain. Later that night, I was not able to feed David again. I thought that if I kept using the nipple shield, I would never be able to latch him on without it, so I decided to start trying to feed him without the nipple shield. By morning I couldn't even latch him on using the shield. I was stressed out and cried at every feeding, which did not help the situation. In the morning, my husband and I rushed to the hospital for the second time. The nurse encouraged me to pump, and I was actually able to pump a couple ounces from each breast. She also managed to latch him on with a shield and told me to feed him that way until he stopped crying. This nurse took one look at my breast and suggested that I make an appointment with my doctor immediately. She thought I had mastitis and suggested nursing on that breast because the baby could suck everything out. My husband took me to my doctor, who explained that I was indeed in the beginning stages of mastitis. He prescribed an antibiotic, told me to keep nursing, and we made an appointment to come back in two days. The entire time that I was on the antibiotic, I kept nursing with a nipple shield. I also tried pumping, but I was only able to get about 1.5 ounces from both breasts. It was clear that the baby was not getting enough food because he would still scream after spending an hour and a half on my breast. We would also put the breast milk that I was able to pump into a syringe and feed it to him, and we also began giving him a couple of ounces of formula using a syringe. I was shocked to see that he could still eat two ounces of formula after nursing for such a long time.

When I came back to see my doctor two days later, I still had a lump, and my breast was still red. I had to come back in a week. During that week, I decided that I would have to stop using a nipple shield if I ever wanted to learn to nurse my baby without it. We hired a lactation consultant to help me at home. Unfortunately, we could not latch him on without the nipple shield. She spent two hours with me and told me to keep going with a nipple shield. She also said that my milk supply might diminish because of the shield, but if this were all I could do, then I shouldn't beat myself up over it.

I continued to use the nipple shield and supplemented with formula, but was still determined to learn to nurse without the shield. So we took our third and final trip to the hospital to get help. This time a third nurse tried to help me. We ended up giving David formula in a cup just to get him to quiet down and then unsuccessfully tried to latch him on without the shield. I then spent about an hour and a half in the lactation consultant's office nursing David with a nipple shield, and she kept telling me that I shouldn't feel bad and that I'm a good mother. What was interesting is that after nursing all this time, we weighed him, and he weighed only two more ounces. He was still hungry and finished the formula.

At this point our family was at the end of our rope, and this stressful breastfeeding experience was starting to have a negative impact on all of us.

My nursing adventure lasted seven very long weeks. My baby was not gaining weight, and he was constantly crying. I gave it all I had, and that is all anyone could possibly do. At the end of all this suffering, we decided to use formula, and he did great after that.

I am not responsible yet

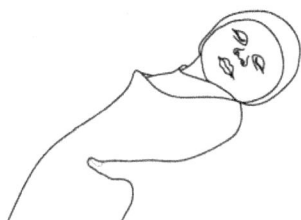

*Raquel, an executive director at a leading professional services firm tells us about her simple delivery and about how much she wanted to nurse her baby. She also tells us about obstacles she faced after a successful delivery. It's a story about how hard it can be to learn to nurse a baby and how important the support of the family can be in order for the mother to succeed. Following this story is another one, also from Raquel, about the birth of her second child. In this story we see what it meant to become pregnant again and give birth again while also caring for a new baby. Interestingly, the second time around, Raquel also had a very difficult time nursing, but like the first time, she persevered.*

The first pangs of labor woke me up in the middle of the night. I felt painful cramps and needed to go to the bathroom several times. At first, my contractions were fifteen minutes apart. I dealt with the pain by lying down with my head in my husband's lap and working through each contraction. I also took a bath several times during this stage of labor. I must have been the cleanest laboring woman around that night. My sister-in-law is an ob-gyn, so I called her to ask how much longer this could go on. She said it could go on for a lot longer and suggested drinking wine and eating. My husband and I followed my sister-in-law's advice, but the dinner was difficult for me. There were times when I needed to stop and just breathe. After dinner, I tried to go to sleep, but I was only able to rest for about two hours. When I woke up the contractions were already seven minutes apart and my body was having a very violent reaction to the food that I ate, and I needed to throw up several times.

I decided it was time to call the doctor even though it was the middle of the night. Unfortunately, my doctor was not on-call at the time, so I spoke with the attending doctor. She asked why I could not wait until it was morning and angrily pointed out that the contractions were not even five minutes apart. I felt I was not doing a good job, and it made my labor seem insignificant, but I was a trooper and waited.

In the morning, I went to the attending doctor's office. My contractions were six minutes apart by then, and I made the smart decision to take my things with me. By the time I got there and was checked in, I was seven centimeters dilated, and the contractions were two minutes apart. The doctor sent me to the hospital immediately. I called my mom and asked her to go to my apartment and to wait for us there. My husband and I really wanted for this to be an experience that only the two of us would share, but since my mom and I are very close, I wanted her to be there when we came back with the baby.

At the hospital, I was sent directly to Labor and Delivery. I am not a screamer, so I groaned a lot and spent a lot of time in a bent position. I wanted an epidural right away, but that didn't happen. It took a while to get me into the system. After I was checked in, I needed an IV and antibiotics because I was Strep B positive. I was not able to move around and had to stay in bed. The wait for the epidural was very long—three excruciating hours. I would throw my leg over the side of the bed and groan because that was all I could do.

Once I had the epidural, I spent five wonderful hours playing cards and relaxing with my husband. Once in a while I would look at the monitor and watch my contractions go by. After five hours the drugs wore off a bit, and I requested more epidural. My son was still not dropping and after another hour the doctor decided to give me Pitocin to speed up labor. I later found out that the doctor was getting ready to do a C-section. The Pitocin helped speed up labor because the next time I was checked, it was clear that my water had already broken and the baby had dropped. I pushed for about twenty-five minutes and delivered vaginally, but with a lot of rips for which I needed stitches. It did not matter, though, because our baby was born! Just before his birth, the doctor needed to suction our baby's mouth a bit because he had passed his first bowel movement inside the womb. In order for the suction to work, I needed to stop pushing. This was actually an interesting point in my labor. We knew that he was coming and that everything was going well, but we were still moments away from birth, so we did not feel responsible for our baby yet.

I was so thrilled with the delivery. I went in with a very simple birth plan—it was to have a baby—and I felt that I followed through with it wonderfully. I had a beautiful baby boy.

I faithfully followed my two sisters' suggestions, which were to get an epidural and to give the baby to the nursery for the first two nights in order to get as much sleep as possible—lots of sleepless nights laid ahead. The hospital staff helped me recover quickly with their attentiveness. The nurses even made sure that I had regular bowel movements—they made me go to the bathroom even though I was scared of the pain and did not want to go.

We tried nursing a bit, and he latched on well, and so breastfeeding started on a good note. Over the next several days, he ate well and the milk started coming. When I returned home, I had some tough times with nursing, but I had a great support team helping me through it. My mom and my sisters encouraged me to continue. My mom would look at a wet diaper and cheer, "See that is a wet diaper, which means that the baby is eating well. This means you are doing a great job!"

Six months after my first baby was born, I got pregnant again. Shortly after, I started spotting blood, and at six weeks, the doctor could not find the heartbeat. She suggested I was miscarrying and asked me to come again at eight weeks to be cleaned out. Naturally, I was destroyed by this news. What was even more traumatizing for me was that my close support group of my sisters and my mom were out of the country at the time. It was the worst week of my pregnancy and my life. But when I came back to my doctor in about a week they found the heartbeat, and I began to cry tears of joy.

After that I did a CVS procedure, which is similar to amniocentesis, and is recommended for late pregnancies. After the procedure, I had to be on bed rest for the next twenty-four hours. Once the test was over, and I learned that the baby had no genetic abnormalities, I was thrilled!

The next few months were difficult because it was hard to be pregnant and to also have a very small child. I was tired: I was working, mothering an infant, and was pregnant all at the same time. My husband was amazing and extremely helpful. He would go on long rides with our son, and this would give me the chance to catch up on my sleep. My son was cute, bubbly, everything made him laugh, and he was good to be around. I knew that I needed to give him as much of my attention and energy as I could.

Another interesting thing about this pregnancy was that I was really stressed out about raising two kids, so my mind became occupied with all sorts of concerns. Where do I put two different kinds of diapers and not mix them up? Where do I put the kid's bath and the infant's bath? I also needed two cribs, two swings, and so on. My sister who had four children and who was very experienced with this sort of stuff came to visit me for the weekend and helped me get organized. But even after that, I was still worried. Somehow I had expected myself to be prepared, but I didn't feel that way. I made my husband gate the kitchen because I was nervous about my older son running off there while I was changing the baby. Of course, what ended up happening was that he would just always want to stay with me and hold the baby's head while I changed him! After the baby came, all of these things that I worried about did not seem to matter that much.

My labor began on the morning of my due date. By the middle of the day, I progressed to contractions that were seven minutes apart. This time I was lucky and my doctor was the one attending. She advised me to come to the hospital. I called my mom, and she came to watch our son. I arrived at the hospital and, just like the first pregnancy, the contractions sped up very quickly, but I was much calmer this time around. My biggest fear in the weeks leading up to labor was that there would be no one to stay with my son, but since my mom was watching him I was calm and could concentrate on my labor.

The situation at the hospital was pretty funny. There was a doctor on-call, and he asked why I was there. I said I needed penicillin for my Strep B and that my doctor told me to come to the hospital. He gave me penicillin and asked if I was going back home. I said, "No, I'm having a baby." He ignored me several times and asked if there was anything more that I would have liked for him to do for me. I asked him to check me, and he said, "Oh my god, you are six centimeters dilated! You are really having this baby!" After this, he called the anesthesiologist and my doctor. Getting the epidural this time was hard. There were several attempts to get it right, and my water was breaking simultaneously. In fact, I only needed a spinal because I was already at nine centimeters. It was great because I could feel the pushing and the pressure but did not feel the contractions. I knew it was going to be my last baby, and I was happy to feel it! My doctor was great; she told me that I was doing so well and that the baby was beautiful. This labor was fast, and it was such a beautiful experience. Every labor should be like this!

I breastfed my second baby for thirteen months. He latched on well. However, he was losing a bit of weight at the beginning, so I did need to supplement with formula. I used cabbage leaves to reduce the engorgement of my breasts, and I think I probably held the leaves for too long and it lowered my milk supply. I had to get it back and that was an incredibly difficult process. I needed to take herbs, and I also got help from a lactation consultant. I almost quit because of how hard it was. It took over my life, but I got the milk back. And then it took about a month to get in sync with my baby and the nursing schedule. He was a hungry baby! He got up every three hours around the clock for six months, and he is still an early riser.

I became a soldier, following orders

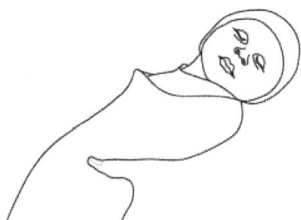

*Denise tells us about the birth of her second child, which turned out to be a stressful experience with worries about pre-term labor and numerous visits to the emergency room. Despite the uncertainly, this mother held on to the hope of a vaginal delivery to a full-term baby. She hoped for a delivery that would be fast and easy. She had an open mind about how the delivery would proceed, but she hoped not to be induced with Pitocin. Denise believed in her doctor and placed trust in her. She could not have foreseen how her labor would progress and with several surprises along the way, the birth of her second child turned out to be an amazing experience.*

*However, labor and delivery was just the beginning of several difficult months that lay ahead. Denise did not plan to nurse her baby unless she felt the baby was very interested in nursing, which he was. The experience of learning to nurse her baby became one of the most enduring things she has ever done in her life. Denise was able to find the inner strength to overcome immense obstacles and was finally able to enjoy nursing her baby.*

The first trimester of my second pregnancy was not eventful. However, the second and third trimesters were more interesting and scarier. I had cervical bleeding twice between twenty-four and twenty-six weeks gestation, and I needed to go to the emergency room both times. Although the bleeding was heavy, nothing was found to be wrong with the baby or the placenta, and I was released to go home. After the second bleeding incident, my doctor suggested I take it very easy. I did not go to the gym, I slowed down my yoga routine, and my husband and I stopped having sexual intercourse. A couple of weeks later, after a long day at the beach and not enough fluids, I began to experience contractions. They were not strong enough to induce labor, but they were persistent. I spent the night in the emergency room and after two IV bags, the contractions finally seized. Following this incident, my husband and I were very worried about pre-term labor. I made sure I had plenty of rest, and I drank water constantly, especially if I felt any contractions. We kept saying that all we cared about was getting to thirty-six weeks, which is what we thought was a big milestone for the fetus.

After all the worry of pre-term labor, my due date came and went. The baby was comfortably head-down, making his usual series of kicks in exactly the same spot, at exactly the same times each day, letting me know that he was perfectly happy. He was growing big inside, and I was growing big on the outside. My doctor sent me to be screened in the hospital for fetal movement and fluids, and since the tests showed nice fetal movements and plenty of fluids, we scheduled an induction for two weeks post due date. One thing that the test showed was that the baby was going to be big. We knew that it is an estimation and in reality the baby could be smaller, but we also knew that the baby could be even bigger. As a last precaution, my doctor ordered a secondary sugar test (I already passed one earlier) to see if I had gestational diabetes and if the baby was getting big because of that. Had the test come back positive, my doctor would have recommended an induction sooner. However, the test came back negative, and so we bought ourselves another week and a half.

The wait was unbearable. Every time I felt something in my abdomen, I would hope that it was labor, but nothing ever materialized. My induction date was coming up in two days. I was very sad, because I knew that induction would be difficult. I knew that Pitocin would bring the contractions on quickly, and my body would not have the time to adjust to their strength. Of course, my very difficult first labor, which lasted more than twenty hours, was always in the back of my mind. I was hoping to have it a bit easier this time around.

As a last resort I decided to get acupressure prenatal massage. The massage was very painful because the pressure points were very sensitive, and the specialist held each point for several minutes at a time. Some points had bruises on them when I got home. I was very tired and went straight to bed.

Early in the morning, I woke from a strange feeling. I felt as though my period had started, and I was leaking. I worried that it was blood again and rushed to the bathroom. I made it to the bathroom (though not to the toilet itself) when I felt water gushing out onto the floor. My water broke! I was ecstatic. Not only because I knew labor was coming soon, but also because I realized that this labor experience may be very different from the last, since last time my water did not break until very late in the game. This made me very optimistic.

I cleaned the bathroom and called my doctor, who told me to come to the hospital. I got ready, told my husband and my older son what was happening, and called my parents to ask them to come over and stay with my son so that my husband could be with me.

At the hospital they confirmed that my water broke, but they also checked and said that there were still plenty of fluids left and that the baby was doing very well. My cervix was closed. Because I needed to be in active labor to be admitted to this particular hospital, I had to go back home. The only way to get into Labor and Delivery without a single contraction would have been to be started on Pitocin, and I did not want to do that.

I went home and stayed in bed for a couple of hours and then called my friend who is also an obstetrician. She was worried. Although she lives and practices in a different state where procedures are different, when she told me that she would never send a patient whose water broke back home, I became very nervous. I called my doctor and told her that I was nervous being at home and not monitored and asked her to think of some way (other than coming in for Pitocin) that she could admit and monitor me. She told me that she needed to think about it, and after a little while she called back with a plan. She said that because my cervix was still closed, she could admit me under the pretext of needing to ripen my cervix (using Cervidil) and asked me if I was okay with that. I certainly was.

My husband and I came to the hospital with everything I thought I would need for labor and for after delivery. The Labor and Delivery room was gorgeous. It was big with a large window and a beautiful view. Maybe when I was in labor for the first time my room was also beautiful. Trouble is, I was already in such pain when I got to the hospital that I hardly remembered my surroundings. Once again, I felt that this time may be different. And again, I felt very optimistic.

A resident doctor inserted Cervidil into my cervix, and after that I needed to stay in bed for two hours to allow the medicine to begin working. I was told that after two hours go by

I was free to walk around so long as they could monitor me for twenty minutes after each hour passed. It was okay for me to be standing up while on the monitor.

I was very calm. I could hear my baby's heartbeat and as I listened to it, I became more and more relaxed. When I was allowed to, I began to walk around. Although I was offered an IV, I did not see a reason for it, so I declined. I sent my husband out to get something to eat and to bring me back some soup, ginger ale, and Gatorade. While he was gone, I began to feel mild contractions.

Over the course of an hour, my contractions sped up and increased in intensity. By the time my husband came back, I was already laboring hard. The contractions were very strong, but there was still a considerable amount of minutes in between, two or three. I chatted with my husband during the downtime and drank fluids. During the contractions I found that leaning on an arm-chair and swaying from side to side while looking out the window helped me get through the pain. The pain, by the way, was becoming more and more intense. It was very different from my first labor. My older son was posterior, so every contraction I felt was in my back and in my hips. This time, the pain was in my lower abdomen. It would grip me hard, so that I had to force-breathe through it, and it would hold for a while, becoming more painful before easing up. This time, I actually understood what breathing through a contraction actually meant. I remember breathing through a contraction and thinking, "Wow, why could I not do this with my first labor?" And then I would remind myself that the worst was yet to come.

My doctor was not on call, but her partner was. I met her previously, and I was comfortable with her delivering my child. To be honest, I was comfortable with pretty much anyone. The experience of labor and delivery is scary the first time around, but is more basic with a second child. I knew that any doctor or resident allowed to practice in my hospital was perfectly capable of delivering my baby. I also knew that the best way to assure that the doctors do their job well is to let them do it. In between contractions I said hello to the doctor who was going to assist my delivery. She told me she would check my dilation in a few minutes and asked me if I had any questions for her. I did not have questions; however, I did remind her that I did not want to have an episiotomy under any circumstances. Shortly after that, she checked me, and I was at five centimeters.

Labor was progressing well, but was incredibly intense. The only feeling I had in between contractions was an urge to have a bowel movement. I made it to the restroom, but realized that I was not able to do it without pushing. Then I realized that this was actually the urge to push.

I was told not to push because I would swell up from pushing before being completely open. Every time a contraction came, the urge to push was stronger and stronger. At this point I was no longer able to breathe through the contractions because I had to control the urge to push. This is when I began to scream through contractions. This was also when the doctor offered to rupture my membrane. At first I declined. I was worried that this intervention was going to somehow complicate my labor. After about twenty minutes of arguing, I realized that I had no idea what I was talking about, and I let the doctor do her job. She ruptured my membrane. If I could score my level of pain at ten before she did that, the score went up to "beyond any scale imaginable" after that.

At this point, the only position I could master was on the bed, on my hands and knees, holding on to the bed rails with my hands. Every time a contraction came and the urge to push followed, I screamed as hard as I could and as strongly as I could to try and divert the energy from my body's natural urge to push down my baby. In between contractions I begged the doctor to check my dilation, but she could not check me too often for fear of an infection. The doctor kept asking me not to scream so loudly; she kept explaining that when it was time to push, I would need my strength to help her deliver the baby's shoulders. She kept reminding me that it was a big baby and that I needed to conserve my energy.

I knew that I was close. But I did not know how close. My strength left me. I felt like I was running, and I could see the finish line, but my legs suddenly went numb, and I could not make them run any longer. I asked for an epidural. Anything, I thought, anything to make this less hard was okay by me. The nurse helped me turn over to my back and started me on the IV.

I needed forty-five minutes on the IV before an epidural could be administered. This last half hour was torture. The pain was so great that I felt as though it was a gigantic force violently roaming inside of me, wanting to get out. In fact, it was only a little baby, and that fact is what kept me going. I tried to look at my husband who was standing over me; his eyes were filled with regret that he could not help me. I tried to think of the moment that I already felt once before, the moment when all pain is gone and only happiness remains and a tiny bundle of warm flesh wiggles against my chest.

The anesthesiologist finally arrived and began to lay out her various instruments in front of me. "Faster," I thought, "please do this faster." She had many questions for me, and I did my best answering all of them. I remember when she asked me whether I had any loose teeth; I said that no, I did not, but wished to say that she may have several loose ones herself if she did not move any quicker. Finally, she was ready and so was I, and, as a last precaution, the doctor decided to check my dilation. To my great surprise she said: "No epidural; she is open," and then all hell broke loose.

In an instant, the room was transformed. Bright lights were turned on, I felt like I was a tooth, about to be closely examined by several dentists. Several other nurses stormed into the room, as if on a cue, and assumed places around my bed. I could barely see my doctor's head poking from between my legs. My husband held my left leg along with a nurse, and two other nurses held my right leg. Another nurse was near the doctor.

I felt a liquid poured over my perineum. My husband later told me that it was iodine. He said that the doctor opened a huge jar of it and spilled it all over the instant my legs were up in the air. Then I heard the magic word: "Push!" I did push, and it felt so great. I thought I was doing such a nice job, but the nurse holding my right leg did not agree. "Don't push with your throat," she said. "That is not where the baby is." After hearing that several times, I finally understood what she was saying. I made it quiet in my throat, I took the strength out of my lungs, and I pushed from my chest and through my abs; I heard: "Good, good, push, push, push…" The next few minutes were a blur. I concentrated on the nurse who held my right leg; I pushed when she said, "push"; I held my breath when she said, "stop"; and when she said, "push" again, I pushed again. I forgot the pain. I forgot when to breathe and how. I became a soldier following orders—I did only what she said and only when she said it.

Suddenly I felt an intense pain, and felt my flesh rip. It was as if a knife split me open, and a burning match was dropped in. And the craziest part of it all was that I don't think I've ever been happier. The head crowned, and I thought, "I did it." Sure enough, a few minutes and a couple more hard pushes later, my baby was born. I did do it. I was in disbelief. I gave birth to a beautiful baby boy, and I felt every minute of it. I was truly happy. It was an amazing feeling of accomplishment and relief. He was adorable, and I felt so blessed to have him. My husband and I held him and smiled.

Although my water broke early in the morning, I was only in active labor for around five hours. My son was born about an hour before midnight. Just to demonstrate the difference between kid number one and kid number two, I have absolutely no idea what his Apgar score was. And I never really bothered to find out; he seemed fine to me. My husband left the room to make calls. He called my mom and asked her to come to the hospital, while my dad stayed home with our older son. Meanwhile, I called two very close friends, let them know that all was well, and asked them to spread the word.

About an hour after delivery, after my placenta was collected for cord blood storage, and I was cleaned up, a nurse helped me get up and use the restroom. I could hardly use my legs, and everything from the waist down was tired and hurt. The nurse helped me put on disposable underwear with two maxi pads. There was a lot of bleeding. Then I was put in a wheelchair, and my swaddled baby was placed on my lap. Triumphantly, I rolled through the empty corridors of the hospital into the maternal recovery wing. I was overjoyed, but I was also solemn. Being a second-time mom, I knew what was ahead. I was bracing myself. Postpartum was just around the corner.

*          *          *

With my first son, I was not able to breastfeed due to a series of events, the anatomy of his mouth, the shape of my breasts and nipples, and poor support from doctors and lactation consultants. My son was brought up on formula, and, although he was a very fussy baby, he was also a healthy one, and grew up to be a healthy and smart boy. When I was pregnant the second time around, I did not think it would be a big deal if I did not breastfeed. I kept telling my friends that I would probably only breastfeed if this baby latched on and just did not let go. To be fair, though, I did go through old breastfeeding books prior to delivery and made any necessary preparation for nursing in the event that I was able to nurse, such as buying a couple of nursing bras, nursing pads, and renting a pump. I also had help from a seasoned breastfeeding mom who sent me some items she found helpful from her experience.

My postpartum room was private, which was a huge change from my first delivery, when I had to share a room and go through another woman and her constantly visiting relatives and friends each time I needed to use the restroom. I was wheeled into the room with my baby and my mom, who had already joined us at that point. We told my husband that he should go home and get some rest; my mom would help me get through the night. My husband did not protest. I took my son in my lap and my mom supported his head. I held my breast with my free hand, putting pressure on the top of the areola to compress it, and my mom directed my son's mouth towards the breast. He took it. And, he did not let go for a long time. My god, he is nursing, I thought. Now this was truly unexpected. These thoughts stayed with me for only a few minutes. Then I realized that I was in as much pain as I had been about two hours before delivery. I called the nurse, and she explained that I was experiencing "afterpains." Afterpains were similar to contractions; they were not so severe that I had to scream, but bad enough that I moaned and could not carry on a conversation. I was amazed at how painful this was considering that I was given high doses of Motrin every six hours. I continued to feel these pains each time my son nursed.

By the middle of the night, I began to feel another kind of pain. This kind would stay with me for a while, as I would later learn, but I did not know this at the time. It was the pain of my nipple being squished flat by my baby's tongue. My nipples were becoming incredibly sore, and I noticed that one nipple was already bleeding. I used lanolin after each feeding, and I wore Lily pads, which had a layer of cool gel on them, to soothe the pain right after nursing. This routine was not helping much, and I knew it was time to see a lactation consultant.

The consultant arrived early the next day and we got to work right away. She first taught me something I thought was trivial but proved incredibly important—how to take my son off the breast. She showed me to take my index finger and insert it just between the corners of his mouth and break the suction. The reason this was important was the fact that I needed to learn to latch him on properly, and that meant putting him on the breast and removing him to fix the latch as often as necessary. I quickly learned that if I did not break the suction, it was nearly impossible to take the baby off the breast without causing myself excruciating pain.

Next we worked on the latch. The lactation consultant pointed out, after observing the baby, that he was tongue-tied. We also both noticed that he had a preference for turning his head to one side only, which meant that a muscle in his neck was tight. Those two issues in his anatomy prevented two very important things from happening. First, he was not relaxed at the breast. His head was not tilted back, and his mouth was not wide open. Instead, his entire body was tight and in a fetal position, and his mouth clamped down on my breast. Second, his tongue had limited mobility; because of this he nursed more on the tip of the nipple and sucked in less breast tissue than he should have to make it more comfortable for me.

Although my baby was wetting diapers, he did not have a bowel movement, which was worrying the doctors. He nursed all the time, and I believed he was certainly getting colustrum from me; otherwise, why would he stay at the breast? But doctors and nurses were not convinced and, of course, there were many suggestions to give him formula. I was told that I would be released from the hospital without my baby if he did not have a bowel movement by the end of the third day. I resorted to giving him a spoonful of formula. Some time later he finally had a bowel movement.

The last day in the hospital, the reality of postpartum set in. I bled a lot, and even though that was a good thing, as I knew I needed to bleed all of that out, it was hard to move without leaving a trail behind. My belly, so round and tight the last few weeks of pregnancy, now resembled a large lump of mozzarella cheese. My back, it turned out, did a lot of work during labor, and so did my inner thighs, and so these parts were in a lot of pain and were very sore. Walking was very hard. A nurse who worked the day shift on the third and last day of my hospital stay came to my bed and said: "I need to see you walk around. Get out of bed. You are not sick." "Easy for you to say," I thought, but followed her advice through the pain and discomfort. Twice up and down the hospital hallway made me out of breath, as if I just climbed up to the sixth floor. "It's okay," I thought. "It is only day three. Patience—I've done this before."

The next two and a half months proved to be the hardest in my life. My nipples became sorer every day until I noticed holes forming in places where cracks used to be. The way in which they subsequently became deformed made me value a phrase my friend and a seasoned nursing mom used to describe her nipples. I had asked her if her nipples ever went back to looking the way they did before nursing. "Well," she replied after a long pause, "they are working nipples." My working nipples started looking like someone very hungry bit off halves of them, and the part that was bitten off never grew back. These open wounds, or "lacerations," as one of my lactation consultants called them, hurt so much that each time my baby nursed I cried. I was in so much pain that everyone around me had to tiptoe when I was nursing, because all of my physical and mental concentration had to be committed to weathering my pain. When I would finish nursing, another type of pain would set in. I developed a condition called "vasospasm of the nipple." My nipple would respond to any change in temperature anywhere on my body, and this would set off a piercing pain that began at the nipple and shot back into the breast tissue, sometimes resonating up in my shoulders and in my back. I had to wrap myself in scarves and sweaters; I constantly had to keep my entire body warm to reduce these spasms.

I saw several lactation consultants and had been seen by a special breast doctor three times. I tried an array of nipple creams, ranging from simple lanolin to a triple-action-all-purpose nipple ointment. The lactation consultants all said the same thing—that my technique was good, but unless I released my son's tongue I would continue to be in pain. The nipple creams did a good job of keeping my wounds soft and stirring away infection, but they were not helping the wounds to close. The pain was severe.

Around five weeks postpartum, I was close to giving up. I kept browsing the Internet for clues as to what I might be doing wrong, but I was coming up with nothing. I finally decided to release my baby's tongue. I was very worried about the procedure but between that and quitting, I chose to give it a try. The procedure was quick, and my son did not cry. The difference, however, was not huge. I noticed a slight improvement, but only slight. I knew that this enhancement alone was not going to get my wounds healed. The next step was committing to a series of sessions with a cranial specialist to work on my son's back, neck, and jaw. Again, I saw slight improvement but not enough to heal. I finally realized that I needed to give my breasts a rest, otherwise they would never heal. I took out the bottles and cranked up the pump.

For a couple of weeks, I pumped almost exclusively and nursed my baby only once or twice a day. My milk supply decreased dramatically, and I sat for hours only getting out a few ounces. Meanwhile, my baby was growing, and he needed more milk. He was also having a much easier time with the bottle, of course, so he ate more than he would have at the breast. I used bottles called "Breastflow," which I liked because they mimicked not only the shape of the areola and nipple, but also the softness of the breast tissue. But even so, I noticed more and more that when I tried to nurse him, he would no longer root for my breast. Finally, one day, he refused the breast altogether. I was devastated. I could not believe that all of the hard work I had put into learning to nurse my baby was in vain.

But I did not give up. I kept putting him on the breast. I realized that I would rather take the pain back than give up nursing him. He resisted at first, but finally, in absence of another source of food, resorted back to my breast. My doctor started me on domperidone, a medication used to increase milk supply. The pain persisted, and the wounds kept oozing blood. It was now week eight, and I wondered how long it would take.

When we came home from the hospital in October, some of the trees outside our windows still had green leaves on them. As I nursed in pain in those first few weeks I thought to myself that it would probably take waiting until all the leaves turned yellow to see my pain improve. Those leaves turned yellow, and orange, and then red, and then fell down to the ground, leaving the branches bare and cold. And still, I was in pain.

It was not until those branches were covered in crispy white snow and my baby was two and a half months old that the wounds finally healed on one breast and then on the other. One day, I caught myself thinking about something I needed to do, some things I needed to buy at the store. To my amazement, I realized that I was thinking this while my baby was nursing. I noticed that there was no pain, no discomfort; in fact I did not feel anything at all. My breast had my baby's mouth on like a glove. The glove moved gently and rhythmically, and at the end of each movement I heard a very reassuring "gulp." "Ah," I thought, "this is it. This is what all these other women describe. I am finally part of this very exclusive and very special club. I, too, can now enjoy my baby's warmth next to my heart, his round, blue eyes staring somewhere far away, his tiny hand stroking my side with a ticklish motion, and these rhythmic, soothing, "haa…gulp, haa…gulp."

Now, at the end of each nursing session, my baby spits out the breast with some milk still on his lips, looks up at me, and cracks up a smile. And as much as I know about the benefits of nursing to the baby, I wonder how much of that is really true and that maybe, just maybe, we mothers made it all up just to enjoy this happy, drunken, milky smile.

I am going to let it go

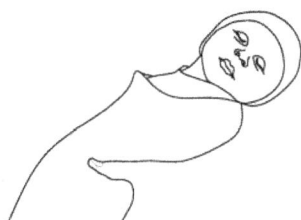

*Suzie, a first-time stay-at-home mom and a production manager, spent a lot of time and effort preparing for a non-medicated birth. She had the right support team and created a home and hospital environment that would help her deliver her baby naturally and without medications for pain relief. Her efforts were not successful because of the very long duration of her labor. She had a choice to make and chose to accept medical help because she realized that she was no longer able to cope with the pain.*

*Suzie's story is important because it shows not only the strength that women need to be successful at non-medicated birth, but also the strength that is required to accept that sometimes things do not work out the way we expect them to. Her story shows the courage of one woman who had to accept a change in the original plan and greet her baby positively, even though his birth was taking a slightly different route.*

During the course of my pregnancy, I paid a lot of attention to developing a birthing plan and preparing for labor. Because I was a recovering alcoholic, I was very careful about any substance entering my body, which meant that I didn't want to have a medicated birth. I had a very well-known birthing coach who recently coached two women through their water births. Through the help of my coach, I focused on strengthening my mind, body, and spirit in order to make sure that I could focus on the task at hand. I made plans to give birth at a birthing center.

One day, I could feel the labor coming. At first, I had contractions that I could eat through. In fact, we went to eat at a restaurant that evening. The following day, the pace of my contractions progressed all the way to being two minutes apart. I went for a swim, but I had to stop during the contractions because I could not talk or move through them. In the meantime, everything was ready upstairs: a birthing ball, drawn shades, the bathtub ready to be filled, and candles ready to be lit. I began to labor at home with my midwife.

After thirty hours of hard work, my midwife checked my progress. I was only one centimeter dilated, and I was in a lot of pain. It was hard to believe that after so many hours and so much pain, I was not opening yet. Late in the evening, I assumed that I would have progressed further, and I decided to go to the birthing center. My mom and my husband went with me. When

I arrived I was checked and, to my dismay, I was told that I was still only one centimeter dilated. I began to cry. I was so upset because I wanted things to go a certain way, but it just wasn't happening. A midwife at the birthing center recommended I take medication for my pain.

I had a choice to make, and I said to myself, "It's okay. I am going to let it go. I am fine with this not working out the way I wanted it to." And I really let go at that point. The midwife needed my body to relax, so she gave me demerol, which made me fall asleep.

In the morning, I was given an epidural and Pitocin to speed up the labor, and soon I was ready to push. Forty minutes later, at the end of the pushing stage, the attending doctor who was delivering my baby did something I was very unhappy about. He said, "You'll either tear, or I'll cut you," and before my husband and I had any time to respond, I was given an episiotomy, which is not a procedure I wanted to have done. What was even worse is that I was incorrectly stitched up. Two months later I was infected and needed to be treated for that. But after all the pain and effort, my baby boy was born.

*    *    *

Before giving birth I had my mind set on breastfeeding, but because I had a breast lift and implants done earlier, breastfeeding was very difficult. My son had problems with the latch, and my milk supply was very low. I tried breastfeeding for about a month, but my son was losing too much weight. The doctor suggested that I gave him formula, and I made the switch. I feel that I should have been warned about the disadvantages of the breast surgery that I had done earlier. I don't think I would have done it if I knew that it would impact my ability to nurse my children later.

If I had to do it again, I would have no problems with having a medicated birth. However, I do regret not being able to create the kind of bond with my son that I could have created if I were able to nurse him. If I do have another child, I would like to try breastfeeding again. Maybe I will be able to organize more support around me that will concentrate on helping me establish milk supply and deal with the types of problems I had with my first child. I also plan to do more research about the impact of the type of surgery I had on breastfeeding and to possibly find helpful information on how to successfully nurse despite it.

This is not a show

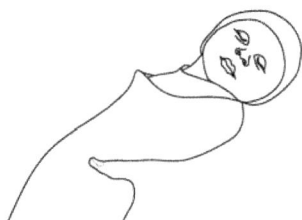

*Jane, a first time mother, did not have a specific agenda when she prepared for her son's birth. The most important thing for her and her husband was to deliver a healthy baby.*

*Jane's story shows emotional issues that a first-time mother and father might be faced with. Jane had extensive family presence before and during her labor, but while she appreciated their support, there were times during her labor when she was not sure it was the right kind of support.*

*Jane's husband was very emotionally involved in the difficulties that Jane was having during labor, and he had to set his emotions aside. After the birth, he was deeply affected by how difficult it was to watch his wife in pain.*

My due date came and went without anything eventful happening. Four days later, mid-morning, I began to feel some light cramps, but I didn't really make much of them because they reminded me of mild menstrual cramps. I kept feeling these light contractions throughout the afternoon, and as the day progressed, they became more painful, but still pretty far apart, so there was no need to go to the hospital. I called my husband to tell him about the situation and encouraged him to finish his day at work. About forty-five minutes later, he ran into the house, ready to go to the hospital. I guess he could not concentrate and wanted to be there to support me.

That evening, my cousin came over to see how I was doing. I remember sitting downstairs in the family room with my mother and my cousin on the opposite sides of the couch watching me as I slid off the couch from the pain. I was trying to pretend as if nothing was happening and actually tried to keep up a conversation. With every contraction, my cousin looked at me with a strange expression on her face and probably thought that she never wanted to go through labor. She eventually realized that this would take a while and left.

In the evening, my contractions became very painful, and I decided to go to the hospital. I wanted to go because I felt that if anything happened to me, I would be safe there. It was quiet on the delivery floor, and it actually felt like I was the only woman in labor there. The nurse came in to check my dilation and announced that I was only two centimeters dilated. I became terrified. If it hurt so much at this point, how much would it hurt later? I was connected to the monitor to make sure everything was going well. After that, I was told to walk around in order to help the labor progress.

Later in the evening, my parents, aunt, and uncle arrived. I remember all of them sitting around the table as I bounced on the birthing ball to relieve my contractions. From time to time, they would turn to look at me with very sympathetic expressions on their faces. I have mixed feelings about the audience-in-the-room experience. On one hand, I'm glad they were there because I felt their support. On the other hand, I thought, "This is not a show. Why is everyone looking at me?"

Eventually my aunt and uncle left, and I was left alone with my husband and my parents. I kept forgetting to do my Lamaze breathing, and at certain times I would just not want to breathe. It was wonderful to have my husband there to remind me not to tense up and to keep breathing. Some time later, an IV was placed. In order to keep moving, we would leave the room, my husband on one side and my father on the other, supporting me and rolling the IV as we walked around the maternity floor. Every few minutes, I would stop and grunt from the pain of the contractions. We walked around for a while, and I eventually wanted to lie down and rest. My husband stayed next to me while I was laboring in bed. I tried to get some sleep since it was the middle of the night, but the contractions were too strong.

During the night, the nurse came in from time to time to check on me. I was still two centimeters dilated and was starting to think the baby would never come out. Early in the morning my doctor gave orders to start me on Pitocin. Finally, when I was five centimeters dilated, my doctor allowed me to get the epidural. I thought the relief would come right away, but no, I had to wait. I recall being in bed, in pain, with my husband on one side and my mother on the other side. I will never forget the expression on my mother's face for as long as I live. She looked so worried and so disturbed. She knew exactly what I was going through and could not handle it, so I asked her to leave, and I think it was the right thing to do for both of us.

The time for the epidural had finally arrived. The anesthesiologist told me to stay on my side, to curve my back, and to remain still. Even today this sounds strange to me. I understood the reasoning behind this, but what a strange request to make of a woman who is in excruciating pain and is having frequent contractions. My husband tells me that I had a mad expression on my face and a crazy look in my eyes. I was tightly holding onto his hand and actually bit him to relieve some of the stress and tension in my body. I guess it was something I needed to do! The epidural was in on the second attempt.

Almost immediately after receiving the epidural, I felt relief. I forgot that I was even in labor, and this is exactly what I was looking for. But, after about thirty minutes, I started feeling some pain again. So I called the nurse and informed her that I could feel my contractions a little bit, and I did not want to feel anything. The nurse told me that was impossible. I was unhappy with her response. I thought that she was acting as if I were just another woman and that nothing extraordinary was happening to me. She did get the anesthesiologist, and I did get a higher dose of epidural, and after that everything was wonderful.

My doctor arrived right when I needed to start pushing. The entire pushing stage lasted about thirty minutes, and I think it was one of the easiest parts because of the epidural. At that particular moment, all I cared about was pushing a healthy, screaming baby out of my body. I needed an episiotomy, but I did not feel the pain of the procedure at all.

The moment our son was born, he was given to me to hold, and shortly after that my husband held him, too. After that, the nurse took him away to do the necessary tests. It was nice to have some time to regroup and realize what was happening. I don't remember our son being gone for too long.

After his birth, I felt extremely happy, energized, and ready to take on the world. Well, at least for the next couple of hours. My husband, however, was absolutely wiped out. He did not have any rest during the entire night and was completely exhausted. It was as if we had given birth together. After a few hours, he went home to call our relatives abroad and to get the rest he needed. He later shared with me how difficult my labor experience was for him. He said he had a hard time staying relaxed while I was in so much pain. He wished he could have transferred the pain, or shared the load, and felt powerless. I can only imagine how difficult it must have been for him.

For a while after the birth of our son, my husband did not want to have more children. He was not ready to watch someone so dear to him struggle with so much again. Luckily, with time, we were both more emotionally prepared, and we did have another wonderful child later.

Prior to giving birth I planned on breastfeeding, and I thought that it was going to happen naturally. I had help with nursing at the hospital, but when I came home I had problems. My baby was not latching on correctly and he was constantly screaming. So I decided to pump for the next couple of weeks, and then we switched to formula.

# The day before Thanksgiving

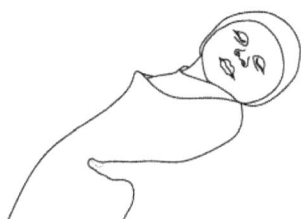

*Natalie, a developer and a stay-at-home mom, wanted to have a vaginal delivery after her first labor resulted in a C-section. Although in the end, Natalie delivered a healthy baby boy, her story shows how difficult it may be to labor when the mother's support team is not being helpful. This is a heart-wrenching story about the struggles of a mother against the medical team which was not helping her make correct choices during delivery.*

Even though I had a C-section with my first child, with my second one I wanted to have a vaginal delivery. My doctor was the same doctor who delivered my first child. In addition, a famous birthing center midwife, in training to become a labor and delivery midwife, was assigned to me by the hospital. As part of the birth plan I worked out with my doctor, the midwife would assist me during labor, identify a time when to call my doctor, and continue to assist us through the delivery.

My contractions began the day before Thanksgiving, early in the morning. I felt a lot of pain and decided to go to the hospital. My midwife checked me, made a sour face, and said that I was not really dilated. She said, "We should really speed this up, because I have a dinner to get to this evening." I was not prepared to hear something like this, and I knew at that point that I had made a mistake in choosing this midwife to help me. Luckily, in addition to my midwife, there was also a resident midwife and a hospital nurse. They were extremely nice and very helpful.

We discussed with my doctor that I would have to be monitored in order to increase my chances of having a successful vaginal delivery after C-section. We also discussed that I wanted to receive an epidural. However, my midwife had different plans for me. She was attending to another labor at the same time as mine, and she also wanted to speed up my labor because she had plans that evening. Thus, she instructed me to be on my feet a lot to make sure labor progressed quickly. I soon realized that the birth plan I worked on with my doctor was not being followed.

As the day progressed, the midwife asked me to use the shower and to stimulate my nipples to progress labor. This was very difficult for me because a bathroom with a shower was not readily available, and I needed to spend time looking for one that I could use. I would have preferred to simply concentrate on my contractions and my breathing instead. In the middle of my search for the shower, I ran into an assistant from my doctor's office. She was incredibly surprised to see me up and about because she knew what my birth plan was supposed to be.

What came next was a heated discussion with my midwife, because she told me that it was time to break my water. Luckily, the resident midwife was there to explain the reasoning for that. She explained that they were worried about the rupturing of the uterus, which is something that can happen if the labor is long and the muscles become increasingly tired. Again, I was shocked that my midwife did not go into any explanation with me and instead told me that because she was in charge of my delivery, I should do what she was suggesting. It turned out that I was five centimeters dilated and that the labor was progressing well. My midwife concluded that indeed there was no need to break my water at that point.

Unfortunately, at the next check up, my midwife did not feel that the labor was continuing to progress well and insisted on breaking my water again. I was so exhausted at that point that I was no longer able to argue with her and allowed this to happen. I also requested an epidural, but my midwife declined, saying that it would slow down my labor. Once my midwife broke my water, she left to attend to her other patient.

Some time went by, and I was transferred to a delivery room. My midwife checked me and told me that it was time to start pushing as I was nine centimeters dilated. She suggested that I should sit on the toilet as I begin the pushing. This was not something I was comfortable with, so I refused. I had no urge to push. In the middle of our argument, my midwife suddenly had to leave. She also took the resident midwife with her. My husband, who had been quietly supporting me this entire time, finally had enough. He was outraged at how I was treated, and he ran after them to have a conversation about what was happening. The midwife's response was that this was not her first labor and that she had thousands of women that she had attended to over the course of her career, and I was just one of them.

It was not until after my delivery that we found out the reason for my midwife's erratic behavior. It turned out that the mother who was laboring at the same time as I had a stillbirth. We realized what a horrific situation that was and, to some degree, came to terms with why she behaved in the way that she did. Still, I felt that I should not have been treated in this way, even though what was happening next door was an incredibly stressful and sad situation. I felt that my midwife should have called my doctor when she knew I was nine centimeters dilated, but she did not, and instead she left to console the family of a stillborn child. Eventually, when she came back, she asked me to push, and again, I had no urge. I did push for about a half hour, after which she checked me again. The resident midwife explained that I had a lip, which, from what I understood, meant that there was something in the way of the baby coming through. I pushed for another hour. Still, no one called my doctor.

Meanwhile, my doctor thought that he should have been called to my labor by now and decided to come and check my progress. He checked me and immediately said, "This baby is not coming out this way!" My midwife replied, "Well, I think this labor is classic. We should let her push further." Hearing this exchange, I had no faith anymore. I was physically drained from pushing. My capillary vessels had popped and my eyes were completely covered with blood. My face was like a bruise. At this point the baby was crowning—you could see the face.

After two and a half hours of pushing, the monitors showed the baby was in distress, and my doctor said that I probably needed a C-section. I couldn't use any breathing techniques because the baby needed as much oxygen as possible. I needed to inhale deep, even breaths if I wanted to make sure my baby came out healthy and without going through an emergency C-section.

Since my midwife did not follow the birthing plan that I had worked out with my doctor and refused to give me an epidural, I now needed to wait for an anesthesiologist before I could have a C-section.

I had to lie down calmly for about forty to fifty minutes in the midst of the most excruciating pain, while simultaneously resisting a now persistent urge to push. Finally, the anesthesiologist was available and so was the operating room. I could not sit up anymore. I was too tired, and they tried to insert the needle while I was lying down. However, I have a very bad back and spine, and it took eight tries before the needle was finally in. The relief was instant. It was the greatest pleasure that I have ever experienced in my life. I was now ready for the C-section.

When my baby boy was born he had a hard time breathing at first and needed to spend two days in intensive care.

My support group was epidural

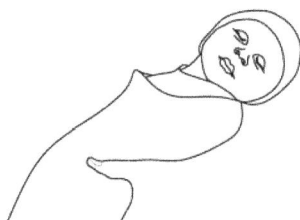

*Linda is a first-time mother, and a medical doctor. Her labor progressed quickly, and although her doctor did not think she would go into labor any time soon, she made the right choice and headed to the hospital.*

*Linda's story demonstrates a fine line between needing pain relief and being able to labor without it. Sometimes, just at the moment when you are ready to give up, you end up at the finish line.*

I finished work and went to see my doctor. She told me that I was still closed and that labor would not begin for a while. She also told me that she was going out of town, and she would see me in a few days! I walked out of her office, called my husband, and said, "I don't care what my doctor says, I'm in labor!"

I crawled home and packed my bag. My husband came from work and said that according to the print-out that I gave him earlier, there were twelve hours in the first stage of labor. He suggested that we relaxed and went for a walk. I responded, "No, let's go straight to the hospital for an epidural!"

We got to the hospital and, of course, they made us wait. I had to put on my ugly face and say, "Hey, I am an attending at this hospital, and I need to be checked right away, and I need an anesthesiologist right away, too."

I was checked and told that I was six centimeters dilated, and this was only three hours after my conversation with my doctor. I was eligible for an epidural, but the only anesthesiologist in the hospital was busy with two emergency C-sections. There was no point in screaming and cursing—I just had to survive. I assumed a position on the toilet—and when I did that, it felt comfortable, so I just stayed there. This helped the mucus plug to come out, and after that I continued to stay in this position for another two hours. My husband, who was walking from the room to the bathroom to check on me, kept telling me, "Relax, honey." I kept replying, "No, honey. Just don't talk to me." At one point, a nurse came in during a contraction, and she was extremely helpful. She asked if I went to any Lamaze classes, and I told her that I had not. She taught me to slowly exhale through each contraction, and that was so helpful that I just kept on breathing this way.

Suddenly, the anesthesiologist rushed in screaming, "Where is this patient who needs the epidural?!" I crawled out of the bathroom, and she said, "Get on the bed quickly because I only have a few minutes." I got on the bed, and they administered it without giving me time to get through the contraction. I immediately felt relieved. The contrast between feeling the pain and not feeling any pain was probably my most positive memory from the labor experience. Epidural was my true support group at that moment; I felt a great sense of relief. What came next was shocking; a resident checked me, and I was nine centimeters dilated. I was disappointed that I was not checked before the epidural! I could have done this without the drugs. Adding to my disappointment was the fact that I needed to lay down for another two hours waiting for the doctor to finish the emergency C-section, while I was fully open!

During the final stage, I felt a little bit of pressure, and I just pushed my daughter out with only five pushes. It was very easy. I only needed a few stitches after the delivery.

My daughter came out with wide-open eyes, and they immediately placed her in my arms. She was very alert and was crying, but stopped once I held her. They asked my husband if he wanted to cut the cord. He said "no," and I said "yes," and then he almost did it in the wrong place! Thankfully, the doctor redirected him.

As for breastfeeding, she latched on right away, and I didn't feel any pain. It felt strange and unusual. The placenta came out right after I began to nurse. I stayed in the hospital for three days, and, since I work there, they gave me a single room at the end of the corridor. It was great; lots of people visited! During the nights, my baby was in the nursery—I felt that these were the last nights that I was not responsible for her, so I took advantage of that and rested.

I was not afraid of my labor

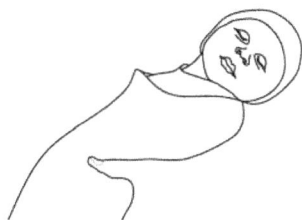

*Jennifer, a first-time mom, chose to have a non-medicated delivery. Her mother's experience—giving birth to six children without epidural— empowered her to think that she could do it without assistance as well. Fortunately for her, labor progressed quickly, and she was not forced to be in pain for too long.*

*An important point to take away from this birth story is how Jennifer approached labor. She did not view it as something that was happening to her, but as something she was doing, something she was in control of. This story underlines the power of the mind in changing the perception of the pain of child birth.*

I wanted to labor without medication because my mother gave birth to six children naturally, and I thought I could do it, too. I also wanted to experience the natural high of Oxytocin that a woman has after delivery, and I knew that being on medication during delivery might interfere with that.

At thirty-two weeks, I learned that my baby was in a transverse position. Every morning I felt her head on my right side, and if she did not turn on her own, I would need to have a C-section. That made me upset because I thought a C-section would make it difficult for me to nurse. My midwife advised me to walk around and to try placing my knees on the couch and bending over with my palms touching the floor. At thirty-six weeks, after all the walking around and trying different positions, the ultrasound confirmed the baby was head-down.

My estimated due date was coming up, and I was almost two weeks past that date, so an induction was scheduled. My midwife did not want me to go past two weeks so that my placenta would not get old. Two days before my scheduled induction, I took a hot shower and felt strange, but I did not experience any contractions. I also had some spicy leftover Indian food. That afternoon, I felt my first contraction, and my next one came five minutes later. My mother told me she did not believe these were real contractions, because she was surprised they were so close together so early during the labor process. She called my husband and asked him to come home. My midwife was also aware of what was happening. I would be getting the midwife who was on-call, and I was lucky to get the one who had been following me during my pregnancy. I think this helped me psychologically.

I did not sit down at all during my contractions. I got into the hot shower with the birthing ball. During the contractions, I stood up and leaned against the wall, and in between, I sat down on the birthing ball.

We went to the hospital in the evening, and after I was checked, I learned that I was only three centimeters dilated. I was surprised, because my contractions were five minutes apart, and I thought I would have been further along. My midwife told me I could either go home, stay in the waiting area, or we could go to the birthing room. I chose the birthing room, and I decided to labor in the shower just like I was doing at home. Hot water relaxed my muscles, and I found that helpful. My midwife was not present with me in the room, and I did not expect her to coach me. We decided not to get a doula because we thought we could do it on our own. During my labor, I depended on my husband and the shower for relief. My mom sat in the corner of the room knitting. My contractions were very painful, and I thought I would labor all night. It felt like the universe was shifting in my stomach. At every contraction I thought maybe I should get an epidural. If I had known it would happen so fast it might have been easier to bear the contractions. I tried to think that contractions were not happening to me, but more like it was me doing something to push the baby out. Standing and pushing against the wall made me feel like I was in control.

After I got out of the shower, they wanted to examine me, and it was the only time I was in bed during my labor. Having to stay in bed made me feel uncomfortable. During the exam, my water broke. I went back in the shower, and while I was in the shower, I started bearing down, pushing. I probably should have left the shower earlier, but I wasn't sure why I was already feeling that and stayed in the shower longer. When I came out, I was shaking, and my mom said I was in transition and went to get my midwife. She came in and said I would be ready for the pushing stage soon because I was fully dilated. My mom was in the room for some time, and then I asked her to leave.

At first, I tried pushing on all fours and on my side. I didn't like that so my midwife suggested squatting. They raised the bed so I held onto the bar and stood on the floor. I squatted during the pushing, and I stood up and rested in between. They placed some towels on the floor. Pushing her out was a strange sensation and felt like I was having a bowel movement. I tried to retain myself at one point, but then I realized that I was actually pushing her out. It would have been nice to be prepared for that feeling. At one point, when I stood up I felt her head between my legs. I could see it was a girl when she came out upside down looking startled. I will never forget the way she looked. Her head crowning was not that painful for me because I was squatting and she came out quickly. Since the bed was still raised, my husband went underneath, and we sat on the floor with our baby.

I put her on the breast right away, and she kind of licked it. Breastfeeding was very difficult at first. It's natural, but it doesn't come naturally. My daughter had trouble latching on correctly, so it was painful the first four weeks, and I cried often. Later, it got easier.

I find it interesting how during my labor I didn't want people around me, but as soon as she was born the Oxytocin kicked in, and I wanted to kiss everyone in the room. I was up all night taking photos and talking to my husband. He was pretty exhausted, though.

After my daughter was born, my midwife told me I was not afraid of my labor. I thought of it as not something that was happening to me, but something I was doing. Standing during labor helped me reinforce that feeling.

The book that influenced my decision to give birth this way was *Active Birth*, which explains that, years ago, women were not forced to lie in bed during their labor and instead gave birth squatting or on all fours.

My daughter was born seven hours after my first contraction, and her birth was exactly how I wanted it to happen.

# Conclusion

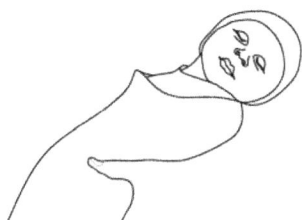

When we sat down to put together the stories in this book, we felt a wave of happiness come over us. Finally, we were able to join many other authors in creating material that can help women go through the challenging and exciting road to motherhood.

Why we did this, what motivated us, is at the same time clear and elusive. On the one hand, there was a need to share our own experience, a need to understand it by asking other women about what they went through. On the other hand, there was a desire to translate the many stories we have heard over the years from our mothers and grandmothers into something more current and tangible. There was a desire to speak to our generation of women about their birthing experiences and to understand what, in our minds, was the most important wisdom that we could carry away from them.

Each time we spoke to a woman and each time we discussed her story, we returned to the same conclusion. It was the inner strength of each woman to face the future, regardless of its type, that guided them to the finish line. It was the emotional and physical desire to push a new life into the world that connected each woman and her story to the next.

The women who graciously shared with us their birthing experiences are now a part of our support group. We recall their wisdom and strength, their fear and fragility, their grace and devotion, as we go about our lives outside of this book, beyond labor and delivery, and even beyond motherhood. We cherish these stories because they remind us about being human, being fearful, and feeling pain, and working hard to overcome those emotional and physical obstacles. These stories remind us about what it is to be a woman.

With much respect and admiration, we thank our contributors for sharing with us the days, hours, and moments of the greatest events in their lives—the births of their children.

# Glossary

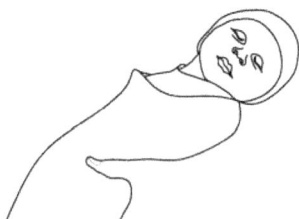

*Abdomen:* The part of the body between the thorax and the pelvis, with the exception of the back; also called belly.

*Active labor:* Your contractions become more frequent, longer, and stronger, and your cervix begins dilating faster—going from three to four centimeters to ten centimeters. In contrast to early labor, you'll no longer be able to talk through the contractions. Toward the end of active labor, your baby may begin to descend, though he might have started to descend earlier or he might not start until the next stage.

*Acupressure prenatal massage:* A massage that uses acupressure points to stimulate the uterus to contract is known to be a way of naturally inducing labor.

*Acupuncture:* An originally Chinese practice of inserting fine needles through the skin at specific points especially to cure disease or relieve pain.

*Amniocentesis:* The surgical insertion of a hollow needle through the abdominal wall and into the uterus of a pregnant female to obtain amniotic fluid, especially to examine the fetal chromosomes for an abnormality and for the determination of gender.

*Amniotic fluid:* Clear fluid in the amniotic sac in which the fetus grows. Cushions the fetus, allows for fetal movement, helps the lungs develop, stabilizes the baby's temperature, and provides a barrier against infection.

*Anesthesia:* Loss of sensation and usually of consciousness, without loss of vital functions, artificially produced by the administration of one or more agents that block the passage of pain impulses along nerve pathways to the brain.

*Anesthesiologist:* A physician specializing in anesthesiology.

*Apgar:* An index used to evaluate the condition of a newborn infant based on a rating of 0, 1, or 2 for each of the five characteristics of color, heart rate, response to stimulation of the sole of the foot, muscle tone, and respiration, with 10 being a perfect score.

*Back labor:* Back labor refers to the intense lower back pain that many women feel during contractions, and some even feel between contractions. This pain is usually attributed to the pressure your baby's head puts on your lower back, but other factors may be at work as well. Back labor has long been thought to be more common when the baby is facing up. But this isn't known for sure. For one thing, ultrasound studies show that practitioners are often mistaken in their assessment of a baby's position, particularly early in labor.

*Bathtub:* During labor take a bath or shower or apply warm compresses or a hot-water bottle to your lower back. Heat may ease the pain and bring you some comfort.

*Bear down:* The urge to push the baby out.

*Birth canal:* The channel formed by the cervix, vagina, and vulva through which the fetus passes during birth.

*Birthing ball:* A large air-filled rubber ball that a woman can sit on during labor. Sitting on the ball encourages a natural swaying or rotating motion of the pelvis, promoting fetal descent. The ball provides perineal support without a lot of pressure and helps keep the fetus aligned in the pelvis. The sitting position assumed on the ball, similar to a squat, opens the pelvis, helping to speed up labor. Gently moving on the ball greatly reduces the pain of contractions. With the ball on the floor or bed, the mother can kneel and lean over the ball, encouraging pelvic motion, which can aid a posterior baby in turning to the correct position, thus allowing labor to progress more quickly. This position is wonderful for a mom who is having back labor caused by a posterior position. The mother's weight is supported entirely by the ball, and the doula or support person has excellent access to the mother's back for massage and counter-pressure.

*Birthing bar* (squat bar): Some hospitals and birth centers have beds with a special attachment called a "squat bar." This bar is used to support the weight of the mother so her legs do not have to if she chooses to squat during labor.

*Birthing center:* Birthing center is a health care facility, staffed by nurse-midwives, midwives, and/or obstetricians, for mothers in labor, who may be assisted by doulas and coaches. By attending laboring mother, doulas can assist the midwives and make the birth easier. The midwives monitor the labor and monitor the well-being of the mother and fetus during the birth. Should additional medical assistance be required, the mother can be transferred to a hospital. Birthing centers are meant for low-risk labors, and do not supersede hospitals. Free-standing birthing centers require hospital backup in case there are complications requiring more complex care. A birthing center presents a more home-like environment than a hospital labor ward, typically with more options during labor: food/drink, music, and the attendance of family and friends if desired. Other characteristics can also include non-institutional furniture, such as queen-sized beds, large enough for both mother and father, and perhaps birthing tubs or showers for water births. The decor is meant to emphasize the normality of birth. In a birthing center, women are free to act more spontaneously during their birth, such as squatting, walking, or performing other postures that assist in labor.

*Birthing coach:* Another name for a doula. A professional trained in helping women cope with pain of non-medicated and/or natural child birth.

*Birthing stool:* A low, U-shaped stool that supports a woman giving birth in a squatting position. It is about the same height as a toilet with an open front. Using a birthing stool allows the pelvic floor muscles to relax, while a squatting position uses gravity to aid the birth.

*Birth plan:* Writing a birth plan gives you an opportunity to think about and discuss with your partner and your health care practitioner how, ideally, you'd like your baby's birth to be handled. Even though there's no way you can control every aspect of labor and delivery, a printed document gives you a place to make your wishes clear. Just remember that you'll need to stay flexible in case something comes up that requires your birth team to depart from your plan.

*Blood glucose:* Keeping blood glucose levels in the normal range is the focus of treatment for gestational diabetes. Gestational diabetes is a form of diabetes found in pregnant women. There is no known specific cause but it is believed the hormones of pregnancy reduce a woman's receptivity to insulin, resulting in high blood sugar. Gestational diabetes affects an estimated two to three percent of pregnant women.

*Blue cohosh:* Blue and black cohosh are roots from two separate plants. The medicinal herbs are used for labor induction. Cohosh is popular among midwives because it is considered a "natural" way to induce labor.

*Bradley Child Birth Class:* This method, developed by American obstetrician Robert Bradley in the late 1940s, embraces the idea that childbirth is a natural process and that, with the right preparation, most women can avoid pain medication and routine interventions during labor and birth. Proponents claim that nearly ninety percent of women who deliver vaginally using the Bradley method do so without drugs.

The program lasts twelve weeks, and is more intensive than other childbirth education classes. The Bradley philosophy argues that it takes months to prepare for childbirth and parenting—mentally, physically, and emotionally—and prides itself on addressing all aspects of natural childbirth, as well as many pregnancy and postpartum issues. The course also emphasizes educating partners to be effective coaches.

*Braxton Hicks contractions:* Relatively painless non-rhythmic contractions of the uterus that occur during pregnancy with increasing frequency over time but are not associated with labor.

*To break one's waters:* To puncture the sac filled with amniotic fluid in which the fetus grows to speed up labor.

*Cabbage leaves:* Some women find that applying cabbage leaf compresses to the breast can be helpful to relieve engorgement. Some believe it is important to limit this treatment because it may also decrease the milk supply.

*Catheter:* A plastic tube that is inserted through a patient's urinary tract into her bladder. A balloon located at the end of the catheter is usually inflated with sterile water to prevent the catheter from slipping out. This is put in place during labor when an epidural is administered (birthing woman is unable to get up to use the restroom).

*Cervidil:* A vaginal suppository, to prepare the cervix for labor; it is used to induce labor.

*Cervix:* The narrow lower or outer end of the uterus.

*Cervix is paper-thin:* When process of effacement has reached one-hundred percent. (As effacement takes place, the cervix then shortens, or effaces, pulling up into the uterus and becoming part of the lower uterine wall. Effacement may be measured in percentages, from zero percent (not effaced at all) to one-hundred percent, which indicates a paper-thin cervix. Effacement is followed by cervical dilation).

*Circumcision:* The cutting off of the foreskin of males that is practiced as a religious rite by Jews and Muslims and as a sanitary measure in modern surgery.

*Codeine:* A morphine derivative that is found in opium; it is weaker in action than morphine.

*Colostrum:* Milk secreted for a few days after delivery and characterized by high protein and antibody content.

*Contraction:* One of usually a series of rhythmic tightening actions of the uterine muscles (as during menstruation or labor).

*CSE:* Combined spinal and epidural anesthesia is a regional anesthetic technique, which combines the benefits of both spinal anesthesia and epidural anesthesia and analgesia. The spinal component gives a rapid onset of a predictable block. The indwelling epidural catheter gives the ability to provide long lasting analgesia and to titrate the dose given to the desired effect.

*C-section (Cesarean section):* Surgical incision of the walls of the abdomen and uterus for delivery of offspring.

*CVS (Chorionic Villus Sampling):* A prenatal test that detects chromosomal abnormalities such as Down syndrome. This is done by analyzing the genetic makeup of cells taken from tiny fingerlike projections on the placenta called the Chorionic Villi. Its main advantage over amniocentesis is that you can have it done earlier—generally between eleven and twelve weeks of pregnancy, although some testing centers will do it at thirteen weeks.

*Demerol:* A fast-acting opioid analgesic drug. Indicated for the treatment of moderate to severe pain, and is delivered as its hydrochloride salt in tablets, as a syrup, or by intramuscular or intravenous injection.

*Dialation:* The expansion of the cervix in labor.

*Doula:* A woman experienced in childbirth who provides advice, information, emotional support, and physical comfort to a mother before, during, and just after childbirth.

*Due date:* This is a date, set by a doctor or midwife and based on the first day of a woman's last menstruation, when a baby's birth is expected. Because the date-setting is not an exact science, the medical term for due date is EDD, or Expected Due Date.

*Echinacea:* The dried rhizome, roots, or other part of any of three composite herbs (Echinacea angustifolia, E. pallida, and E. purpurea), that are now used primarily in dietary supplements and herbal remedies, and that are held to stimulate the immune system.

*Effaced (Effacement):* The shortening, or thinning, of the cervix before or during early labor. Prior to effacement, the cervix is like a long bottleneck, usually about four centimeters in length. Throughout pregnancy, the cervix is tightly closed and protected by a plug of mucus. When the cervix effaces, the mucus plug is loosened and passes out of the vagina. The mucus may be tinged with blood and the passage of the mucus plug is called bloody show (or simply "show"). As effacement takes place, the cervix then shortens, or effaces, pulling up into the uterus and becoming part of the lower uterine wall. Effacement may be measured in percentages, from zero percent (not effaced at all) to one-hundred percent, which indicates a paper-thin cervix. Effacement is followed by cervical dilation.

*Emergency C-Sections:* A C-section that is not scheduled and is performed when an unforeseen complication arises during labor.


*Engorgement:* Breast engorgement occurs in the mammary glands when too much breast milk is contained within them. It is caused by insufficient breastfeeding and/or blocked milk ducts. When engorged, the breasts may swell, throb, and cause mild to extreme pain. Engorgement may lead to mastitis (inflammation of the breast), and untreated engorgement puts pressure on the milk ducts, often causing a plugged duct. The woman will often feel a lump in one part of the breast, and the skin in that area may be red and/or warm. If it continues unchecked, the plugged duct can become a breast infection, at which point she may have fever or flu-like symptoms.

Though it may seem natural to decrease breastfeeding, it is important to continue to reduce the levels of milk. It is, in fact, generally beneficial to breastfeed very often to keep the breasts relatively empty (a lactating breast is never really empty).

Treatment for engorgement, plugged ducts, and infections all include frequent nursing to empty the breast. Application of wet heat and gentle massage (from the part(s) of the breast that are engorged or lumpy toward the nipple) right before nursing often helps, as well. Nursing with the baby's chin (the "moving part" of the baby's mouth) pointed toward the worst-affected part can also help clear it up.

If the problem has developed to the point of mastitis, care to eat and drink enough and well enough can help. Bed rest and frequent nursing (no longer than two hours from the beginning of one feeding to the beginning of the next) are important. An untreated (or ineffectively treated) breast infection can develop into a breast abscess, which may require surgical draining. A breast infection that continues for more than twenty-four hours or gets severe should be reported to the woman's doctor; she may need antibiotics.


*Epidural (anesthesia):* Anesthesia administered to a laboring mother into the epidural space at the base of the spine to numb the lower body. It decreases or eliminates pain, enabling her to save her strength for pushing. It can numb the lower body entirely, so she's unable to feel contractions when it is time to push out the baby.

*Episiotomy:* An incision in the perineum (the area between the vagina and the anus) to enlarge the vaginal opening and prevent tearing during delivery.

*Evening primrose oil:* Contains ingredients that your body can use to produce a hormone called prostaglandin. This hormone is believed to be the precursor to the Oxytocin hormone that makes the uterus contract. It is theorized that the body will absorb these ingredients and produce prostiglandins earlier, causing the cervix to ripen, which may (or may not) initiate the production of Oxytocin that starts the labor.

*Fentanyl:* An opioid analgesic, first synthesized by Janssen Pharmaceutica (Belgium) in the late 1950s, with an analgesic potency of about eighty times that of morphine. Fentanyls are extensively used for anesthesia and analgesia, most often in the operating room and intensive care unit.

*Final stage:* Pushing the baby out.

*Forty-two weeks (42) (Gestation):* The period of time a baby is carried in the uterus; full-term gestation is between 38 and forty-two weeks (counted from the first day of the last menstrual period).

*Hand-held Doppler:* The Doppler transmits the sounds of your baby's heart rate either through a speaker or into ear pieces, and it's a popular option for low-risk pregnancies and for mothers who choose not to have an epidural and do not need to have labor induced. It's non-invasive, easy to use, and portable. It allows laboring moms to wander the halls, take a shower, and stay mobile for as long as possible.

*Heart murmur:* An atypical sound of the heart typically indicating a functional or structural abnormality.

*Homeopathic remedies:* Remedies that are part of a system of medical practice (homeopathy) that treat the disease (problem) especially by the administration of minute doses of a remedy that would in healthy persons produce symptoms similar to those of the disease.

*Hypertension:* Abnormally high arterial blood pressure. Patients with this condition need to be closely monitored while pregnant.

*Hypnobirthing:* Consists of a series of relaxation techniques used to help laboring mothers decrease pain and emotional stress during childbirth, without the use of drugs. It is a form of self-hypnosis used primarily during a non-medicated vaginal birth.

*Incision:* A cut or wound of body tissue made especially in surgery.

*Induction:* The act of causing or bringing on labor.

*IV:* An apparatus used to administer a fluid (as of medication, blood, or nutrients) intravenously.

*Labor and Delivery (place):* A room designed to accommodate a woman's labor, delivery, and recovery.

*Labor down:* Refers to the mother's body pressing the baby down into her birth canal without her voluntary effort of pushing. The mother may be breathing or grunting slightly during contractions but she is simply allowing her body to do the pushing without physically bearing down.


*Lactation consultant:* A lactation consultant is a health care provider recognized as an expert in the fields of human lactation and breastfeeding. A Board Certified Lactation Consultant will have the initials IBCLC after her name.

*La Leche League:* La Leche League International (LLLI) is an international non-profit organization founded in 1956 in the USA to give support and information to women who choose to breastfeed their babies. It encourages breastfeeding on cue from birth onwards, and continuing for as long as desired by the mother and child.


*Latch:* In breastfeeding, "latch" refers to the positioning of the baby's mouth on the mother's breast.


*Lip (Anterior Cervical Lip):* A condition in labor during which part of the cervix does not dilate at the same rate as the rest of it. This creates an obstruction, and it becomes harder to push the baby through.


*Local anesthetic:* An anesthetic for use on a limited and usually superficial area of the body.


*Lochia:* A discharge from the uterus and vagina following delivery.


*Mastitis:* An infection of a milk duct in the breast, most commonly between ten and twenty-eight days after delivery. Symptoms include swelling, tenderness, redness, and fever; treated with antibiotics.

*Meconium:* A dark greenish mass of desquamated cells, mucus, and bile that accumulates in the bowel of a fetus and is typically discharged shortly after birth.

*Midwife:* A person who assists women in childbirth.

*Milk ducts:* Also know as Lactiferous ducts. These are lobes of the mammary gland at the tip of the nipple. They are also referred to as galactophores, galactophorous ducts, mammary ducts, and mamillary ducts.

*Misoprostol:* A medication administered in order to induce labor by softening the cervix.

*Monitor:* A device for observing or measuring a biologically important condition or function.

*Monitor by hand:* When the practitioner assesses the mother's contractions by laying his or her hands on the mother's belly.

*Mucus or mucus plug:* A collection of mucus, often tinged with blood, that blocks the cervix during pregnancy; known as the "bloody show" when discharged prior to labor. The texture and amount of mucus discharged varies greatly from woman to woman.

*Narcotic:* A drug (as codeine, methadone, or morphine) that in moderate doses dulls the senses, relieves pain, and induces profound sleep.

*Natural birth:* Natural childbirth is a childbirth philosophy that attempts to minimize medical intervention, particularly the use of anesthetic medications and surgical interventions, such as episiotomies, forceps and ventouse deliveries, and C-sections.

*Nipple shield:* A nipple shield is a nipple-shaped sheath worn over the areola and nipple during breastfeeding. It is typically used if the baby won't latch to the nipple itself.

*Nubaine:* Nalbuphine (Nalbuphine Hydrochloride) is a synthetic opioid used commercially as an analgesic under a variety of trade names, including Nubain. It is noteworthy in part for the fact that at low dosages, it is found much more effective by women than by men, and may even increase pain in men, leading to its discontinuation in the UK in 2003. Nalbuphine is a potent analgesic. Its analgesic potency is essentially equivalent to that of morphine on a milligram basis. Its onset of action occurs within two to three minutes after intravenous administration, and in less than fifteen minutes following subcutaneous or intramuscular injection. The plasma half-life of Nalbuphine is five hours, and in clinical studies the duration of analgesic activity has been reported to range from three to six hours.

*Nurse-Midwife:* A registered nurse with additional training as a midwife who is certified to deliver infants and provide prenatal and postpartum care, newborn care, and some routine care (as gynecological exams) of women.

*Ob-gyn:* A physician who specializes in obstetrics and gynecology.

*Perineal tears:* Tears in the diamond-shaped area on the inferior surface of the trunk which includes the anus and the vagina.

*Phenergan:* Promethazine is a first-generation H1 receptor antagonist antihistamine and antiemetic medication. It is a prescription drug in the United States, but is available over the counter in the United Kingdom, Switzerland, and many other countries (brand names Phenergan®, Promethegan®, Romergan).

*Promethazine:* A strong anticholinergic with sedative effects.

*Pitocin:* A synthetic version of Oxytocin used especially to initiate or increase uterine contractions (as in the induction of labor).

*Placenta:* A pancake-shaped organ that develops in the uterus just twelve days after conception, providing nutrients for the fetus and eliminating its waste products. It is commonly referred to as the afterbirth because it's delivered after the baby.

*Placenta Previa / Low-lying placenta:* A pregnancy-related condition in which the placenta is attached too low on the uterine wall, fully or partially covering the opening of the uterus. The condition can cause hemorrhaging in late pregnancy or make vaginal delivery impossible.

*Post date:* Any date after the estimated delivery date (forty weeks).

*Postpartum:* The period following the process of giving birth to offspring.

*Postpartum hemorrhage:* A copious discharge of blood from the blood vessels after the process of giving birth to offspring.

*Post-term:* When pregnancy lasts beyond forty-two weeks.

*Ripen the cervix:* To ripen the cervix is to help prepare the cervix for labor. There are numerous ways to achieve this.

*Rocking chair:* A chair with two curved bands of wood (also know as rockers) attached to the bottom of the legs (one on the left two legs and one on the right two legs). Many find rocking chairs soothing because of the gentle rocking.

*Sonogram:* An image produced by ultrasound.

*Stadol:* A narcotic pain reliever commonly used during labor and delivery.

*Stress test:* This test records the fetal heart rate in response to induced mild contractions of the uterus.

*Suctioned:* To remove from a body cavity or passage by suction.

*To be cleaned out:* To have an abortion.

*Tone the uterus:* The uterus is a major female reproductive organ. One end, the cervix, opens into the vagina; the other is connected on both sides to the fallopian tubes. Toning the uterus means helping to cause the pre-labor contractions that help a woman's uterus to prepare for delivery.

*Uterus:* The hollow, pear-shaped organ in which a baby grows. During pregnancy, the fist-sized uterus goes from weighing about 2 oz. to weighing about 2.5 lb. and holding a baby.

*VBAC:* The vaginal birth of a baby after a woman has already had a child by cesarean. While VBACs are increasingly considered a safe option, an estimated one percent of women attempting this will have a uterine rupture and require an emergency cesarean.

Some definitions from the Glossary have been taken from the following websites:

www.womenshealthmatters.com

www.babycenter.com

www.MedlinePlus.com

www.pregnancytoday.com

www.wikipedia.org

www.pregnancychildbirth.com

www.midwifeinfo.com

www.birthingnaturally.net

www.ingramcontent.com/pod-product-compliance
Lightning Source LLC
Chambersburg PA
CBHW060900280326
41934CB00007B/1128